# Born from Kidney TRANSPLANT mother

Dr. Kesorn Pechrach Weaver

# Born from Kidney TRANSPLANT mother

Dr. Kesorn Pechrach Weaver

Pechrach Publishing
**England**

# Born from Kidney Transplant Mother
By Dr Kesorn Pechrach Weaver

**ISBN 978-0-9931178-4-8**

**PECHRACH PUBLISHING**
7 Boundary Road, Bishops Stortford, Hertfordshire, CM23 5LE, England, United Kingdom. Tel: (+44) 1279 508020, +44(0) 7779913907, +44(0)7443426937

Published 2016 by Pechrach Publishing

*This book is dedicated to my son,*

*Neran Jame Pechrach Weaver.*

# Introduction

When I was pregnant as a kidney transplant mother, I try to research and find out information about the pregnancy and kidney transplant mother. Unfortunately, I found nothing much and nothing is answer my questions. After I lost my first pregnancy, I have no concerned because I had been reassured it is common for general woman.

However, when I lost the second pregnancy with stillbirth at 23 weeks and 5 days, I know it is not common anymore. I started to find out more about my immunisation medicine that I took during my pregnancy, what are they affect to the baby in the womb, how damage of my kidney transplant during pregnancy and outcome of the baby after birth. Again, I was disappointed and nobody can answer those questions.

With my third pregnancy, I started to keep records of documents, keep close eyes on my health, my kidney transplant and my pregnancy. As we have known, only one kidney transplant has to work for myself and for the baby inside my womb. It has to work harder for two people than only one. The bigger the baby, the harder it works.

The delivery time is set when the health of the kidney transplant alarm with the high blood pressure, which could damage her internal organ and lost her transplant kidney function forever. Therefore, it would be on the safe side to deliver the baby while the health of the kidney transplant mother still has no too much harm done. It is in the win-win situation.

Although the baby was born premature, the consultants and doctors would make sure it can survive with the help of the premature baby unit, SCABU and NICU. At the beginning the premature baby would look so small compared to a full term baby. However, by the time when they are two years old, they would look the same and could not see the difference between them.

I hope this book will shed some light to the kidney transplant woman who wish to have her own baby to prepare her mind and her body. To learn from my experience about what process she will go through and what is the outcome could be happening. I wish I had ad read this book when I started my family and got pregnant.

Dr. Kesorn Pechrach Weaver

15 January 2016

England, UK

# Acknowledgments

I would like to thank my beautiful son, Neran J. Pechrach Weaver and my amazing husband, Dr. P. M. Weaver for enthusiasm advice, suggestion and non-stop supporter while I was writing this book.

Many Thanks to my awesome family in Thailand for their continuous support, understanding and encouragement.

Special thanks to my kidney donor sister: Miss Somjan Pechrach for giving me a new life and opportunity to distribute this knowledge to mankind.

My best friends Rajiya Sultana, Anna Wlodarczyk and Kanae Jinkerson for their cheerfully support.

Thanks to Prof. J.W. McBride, Prof. J. Swingler, Prof. Suleiman M Sharkh, Peter Wheeler and Peter Wilkes for their support while I was in the end stage kidney failure.

Thank you to Mr Christoph Lees, Dr Kate Farrer, Miss Fatemeh Hoveyda, Dr Peter Yeh, Dr Amanda Ogilvy-Stuart, Dr H Wong, Lynne Radbone, Tina Pollard, Miss Charlotte Patient, Dr Lisa Willcocks, Dr David Jayne, Mr G A Hackett, Dr John Bradley,

Dr Edile Murdoch, Dr J S Ahluwalia, Dr A Curley, Dr A D D'Amore, Dr A W Kelsall, Dr G Ng, Dr N Yeaney, Dr Jagjit Takhar, Dr Pritpal Takhar, Sisi Oo, Jan Graves, Jill Wisbey, and Michelle Ford.

Finally, I would like to thank the professional, specialists, medical staffs in Rosie hospitals, Addenbrook hospitals, Portsmouth hospitals and Parsonage Lane Surgery.

# Table of Contents

# Table of Figures

# List of Tables

# Chapter 1

# Transplant Mother

## End stage kidney failure

I have a kidney transplant in December 2002 during Christmas celebration. I had nephrotic syndrome as a child. I have undergone a renal transplant for glomerulonephritis in Portsmouth. My sister flew over to the UK and prepares to process the matching. She donates one of her kidney to me. She has to pass enormous tests includes physical test, mentality test and psychology tests. The tests have been repeated again and again before we are finally in the same theatre.

At that time it must be a good deal for topic of selling human organs in the dark market. The transplant coordinators have to try very hard to prevent the case happen in their hospitals.

I was 33 years old when I was diagnosed with end stage kidney failure. I was very shocked and not believe of the doctors' test results. That is because I was the scientist myself. I do a lot of experiments and I know there are gaps of error happen in every test. I try to ask them to repeat the kidney function test again and again.

Not only my surprising, but also for them as well. How can an end stage kidney patient who kidney function less than 7% live normal life? The answer is simple, it is because of my body used to it, the body adapts to its own system with less functionality.

At that time I was a PhD student in the Electromechanical Research Group, University of Southampton, United Kingdom. As an electrical engineer with many years experience in the design and construction of electrical system both commercial and industrial plants. I have never released nor have any question with my health at all. I eat, sleep, get up and work just like other people do.

# Dialysis

It looks me more than 2 months to finally accept the options they offer to me about what to do with my life.

**Option 1:** if I do not want to do anything with my body, my kidney will work less and less. Finally, the system will shut down. I will feel tired, more tired and get to the sleep stage and die peacefully. They cannot specify how long I will live until that day.

**Option 2:** Start dialysis, which it can be haemodialysis or peritoneal dialysis.

- Haemodialysis

- Peritoneal dialysis

**Option 3:** Kidney transplants. I would put on the waiting list to receive organ donation. In my case it would be more difficult than others because my race is from an Asian. It is not a lot of Asian people in this country. Most of organ mostly from the accidents from the car crash which the brain dead.

It is an option but they have no idea how long I have to wait from since it is not only I am in the queue but also if the donated organ is matching or not. If it is matched other patients more than me, it has to go to others.

The last option is, live donor. This usually comes from a close family, parents, sister-brother and close relatives. It is a high chance to find matches in the same DNA than general people.

# Kidney Transplant

Most people who need a kidney transplant are able to have one, regardless of their age, as long as they are well enough to withstand the effects of surgery. The transplant has a relatively good chance of success

The person is willing to comply with the recommended treatments required after the transplant – such as taking immunosuppressant medication and attending regular follow-up appointments.

Reasons why it may not be safe or effective to perform a transplant include having an ongoing infection (this will need to be treated first), heart disease, liver failure, cancer that has spread to several places in your body (metastatic cancer), and AIDS (the final and most serious stage of an HIV infection).

However, people who have HIV that is being effectively controlled with medication can often have a kidney transplant.

# Matching Process

My sister and I have lived together for 6 months while she has to do exercise and look after me while I was on dialysis.

Unlike many other types of organ donation, it is possible to donate a kidney while you are alive because you only need one kidney to survive. This is known as a living donation.

People who want to be considered as a kidney donor are tested very carefully to ensure they are a suitable donor and are fit for the operation needed to remove a kidney.

Ideally, living donations will come from a close relative because they are more likely to share the same tissue type and blood group as the recipient, which reduces the risk of the body rejecting the kidney. However, donations from those who are not blood relatives are sometimes possible.

Kidney donations are also possible for people who have recently died. This is known as deceased kidney donation. However, this type of kidney donation has a slightly lower chance of long-term successes on dialysis.

# The Transplant Procedure

The transplant receives a kidney from a living donor, this will be a carefully planned operation.

You will then have surgery to insert the new kidney and connect it to your blood vessels and bladder. The new kidney will be placed in the lower part of your abdomen (tummy). Your own kidneys will usually be left in place.

A kidney transplant is a major surgical procedure with a wide range of potential risks. In the short term, these risks include blood clots and infection. Longer term problems, which include diabetes and an increased risk of infections, are usually related to the immunosuppressant medication that needs to be taken continuously to reduce the chance of rejection.

Because of the risk of further problems, people who have had a kidney transplant require regular checkups for the rest of their life.

# Change of Medication

The process to be ready for pregnancy, the suppress immunization medication has to be safe for baby. Therefore, the period of the recent change type of medicine over, I have to see the renal consultants to check my Creatinine and other kidney function whether it is responding well to the new medication.

This will take about 6 months. In the beginning I will go to the clinic every two weeks, a month, two months and three months. I have to wait the renal consultants are happy with my kidney function with new blood and overall health check results before they can give me a green light to go ahead for the baby plan.

Born from Kidney Transplant Mother

# Chapter 2

# 1st Pregnancy: Miscarriage

I was so exciting to see 2 lines on the pregnancy test. TO make sure, I do another test and the results are the same.

It is quite exactly as our plan. When we decide to have a family and to a new member add to our family. Our baby is the most favorite for every couple. We have been married for a year and my transplanted kidney is working excellent. My Creatinine is in the good range. My condition is stable.

I have consulted with my renal consultant and I receive the green light to go for it. However, I have not known any transplant woman in our hospital have a baby after kidney transplant at all. I asked my renal consultants, but have not got any answers. It may be they want privacy or nobody wants to talk about it. As we all know only one kidney to save our life in order for us to live normally still hard, don't you dare to think about support another person's life.

I try to search the internet, read some research about pregnancy in kidney transplant. However, I cannot find anything really relate to the topic, I am looking for. It may be because a number of women have a transplant is less or a number of women who at the age of productive is less or transplant woman who at the age of able to produce and be healthy enough to try for a baby is less or whatever. As we always know that most of kidney end stage failure before transplant, some develop from diabetic before progressing to kidney failure. Also, it can go in another direction of having a kidney disease first and progress to others.

# First Month

Every minute after I learn that I pregnant, I look after myself very well, I eat fruits and vegetable. I start to drink soy milk because I cannot drink the cow milk. It upset my stomach. I always have diarrhea after I drink it just a few minutes later.

With no family support in the foreign country, the person I rely on most is my husband. We talk and discuss everything together. Most of my friends I know I always see them pregnant and 9 months later they have a baby. It seems simple like that.

# Second Month

Nothing changes much in my body except I eat more and sleep more. I feel sick in the morning same day, but not every day. I still take my anti-rejection as usual. My GP prescript a new medicine to aid in it is called folic acid. They said it will help the baby to develop the spinal core. It starts to form every early age as early as 4 weeks. Then, the early as knowing that we are pregnant, we should ask the GP and ask for folic acid. This is a new knowledge for me.

# Third Month

Roughly about 12-13 Weeks, it is approximately. It is the first appointment I have to go to the ultrasound scan unit. It has been booked advance by the GP over 4 weeks since they know each woman schedule.

The waiting area is full of couples; Most of them are daddy to be and a mummy to be. Some woman may come with her mother in case her husband or her partner is not available. This is the first scan, most couples are so excited to hear the heartbeat and see the picture of the little one inside the mother's womb.

The book schedule is always late. It is not always on time. I do understand because it is a human working on another human. It is not robots which will see the same thing at the same position. Some of the fetus may be on the left or right, have to find it. Some of them are hidden very well. It takes a scanner graphed for a while to find it.

When it is my turn, I was asked to lie down on the bed. The scenographer set her computer to be ready to show the picture of the frequency wave. She put the gel on the probe. She moves the probe all over my lower stomach areas, slides the probe to the left, right, up and down. After she did her profession job for quite a long time, she asked her college to join for a second opinion. I still have no idea what happen here. I still think this is the normal procedure.

She second scangrapher seem like more experience than the first one ask my permission if she will use another probe to do internal scan because the external probe scan over my stomach is not sensitive enough in the case of the fetus is younger than we are expecting. The Internal probe will be able to detect the heartbeat sound better than the external one.

I have no objection at all. She then plans a smaller probe cover with and insert inside. After for a while, she has done or of checking and told me they were finished the job. They ask my husband and me to wait in another room. When I come out the waiting room is quite an entry. We must be in the scan room for ages.

While we are waiting in the room, one of the obstetricians comes to talk to us with some of the documents about miscarriage. At that time I had no idea at all what is about. I have never heard about it before. Then, she explains about how the baby was developing as it should be. Or it may be because of the chromosome, or DNA is not right. Therefore, it is sop growing. She also added it is normal for general woman as well. Not only happened to the kidney transplant woman. She shows us the percentage of miscarriage in the world. I would explain my feeling as numb. I cannot feel anything; my brain does not accept what she told us. I believe they are wrong; the baby may be too young for them to detect it with any tools.

# Miscarriage

However, she gives us 2 options:

First Option: wait for a few weeks, the lump of blood should come out itself. It is the nature of expelling waste from our body. It is just like a period which woman has it every month. However, this may be dangerous of the blood keep coming without stopping. My body will lose a lot of blood and make my faith or create complicated later.

Second option: They will schedule induce procedure which this method should be safer because it have done in the hospital under specialist. They will make sure that I am fine and the blood stopped before letting me go home. I should live a normal life after that.

The Obstetrician is very kind; she has urged us not to make a decision like now. She said go home and have thought about it. If I want to go for the first option, I do not have to do anything. However, if I want to start my new life straight always, I can give a call. They will set the date to start the procedure.

# At Home

I could not sleep at all. I feel tired, but my eyes just not close. My brain keeps running round and round like the halt hard disk. My mind always says no, I don't believe it.  Again, I do a lot of research about miscarriage. I am in deep of the knowledge about this topic more than my PhD degree in engineering. I can say it is hard to talk about this with other people. It looks like something is wrong with me. I feel like it is my mistake, but I have done nothing wrong to have it happen.

I cannot blame anybody and I cannot blame myself as well. My feeling, I just want to hide it from the outside world. I remember I did not leave my house for two days after my husband goes to work, I close the curtain down. Stay quietly by myself. I still hope for a miracle to happen. I wish the obstetrician was wrong, the ultrasound scan was wrong. On the third day, I called my sister who donated one of her kidneys to me and also she is a nurse for more than 20 years, I told her the whole story. She told me it was life and nature. At this point I use my brain instead of my heart. I give a hospital a call. I choose the way of my life and I do not want to wait. I have to wait for another 6 months to try for a baby again.

# At the Hospital

When we arrive with a small bag of clothes, toiletries, books and a laptop, the whole ward is empty, no staff and no patients. It is very quiet; I can hear the pin drop. We sat for a while to settle. My hospital and I am the second home since I was an end stage kidney failure patient. A young nurse comes to explain the procedure, what will happen to my body, what complicated it can be, and what can go wrong. However, as she explains, she tries to reassure that she has experienced and they have doctors ready for every situation.

Why do I have to pack my bag? Since I was a kidney transplant patient who has to do the procedure of miscarriage, If in case of complicated, I may have to stay overnight at the hospital. However, if anything goes as planned, I should go home after few hours.

# Induce Procedure

She gives me two tablets; it is to insert called Pessaries that are inserted directly into your vagina, where they dissolve.

While I lay down in my bed and my husband sit next to me and working on his computer have experienced symptoms similar to a heavy period, cramping and heavy vaginal bleeding. I have to lie down without moving for a couple hours. This is to make sure that bleed is stopped. I feel empty, my eyes look at the white ceiling, my brain stop thinking and my heart ache.

I just understand now why the whole ward and the whole wing is no patients, which it is different from other wards where they run out of bed and extremely busy. This procedure is heart broken, nobody wants to come here. The nurse asked me to ring the hospital if the bleeding becomes very heavy.

I allow going home in the afternoon on that day after the miscarriage procedure is completed. My husband drives and stayed quietly all the way back home.

Born from Kidney Transplant Mother

# Chapter 3

# 2nd Pregnancy: Stillbirth

We have to wait for 6 months for my health, my body and my soul to be ready before we can try for another baby. However, we get it straight away. I don't know if we are lucky or I do a good calculator about my egg time. Now I know about the risk of being miscarried. This time we keep quiet about the news to ourselves, which was different from the previous one that we told friends and family strange way when we knew the news.

## 12 Weeks

The process of the second pregnancy is the same as previous. I inform my GP as soon as I know my pregnancy test results. Again, he gave a prescript to me with folic acid immediate with the same reason of the spina construction. The midwife has been informed as well as the hospital.

When the 12 weeks arrives, this time we prepare more than the last time about the in case of "no heartbeat" from the ultrasound scan result. I receive the booking appointment and time slot to see the consultants. This time we are the last queue, I do understand why they have to put us in the last. I guess because we have a bit of history.

I would say that I could not sleep from the night before. It is impossible at all to detect a heartbeat, although there are some advertise about the instruments which on the market say that they can listen to the baby's heartbeat. However, the ages of the fetus must be older than three months or many certain weeks.

I tell myself if the ultrasound scan results cannot find the baby heart beat again. I would accept it easier. It would not be shocked like the last time.

Wow! Just only the scangrapher put the probe cover with the clear gel on top of my stomach. The heart beat sound echoes out from the speakers so loud. It was amazing sound ever in the world that I have ever heard. This sound shows the sign of life. She prints me some picture. It's just a small core shape like a bean a small bean. She said its size 1-2 CM with a heart.

We are so happy this time. We tell our friends and family after we get the scan results and know it is alive and it is there inside me. This time I do everything as it says in the books about food, exercise, and I can't eat such as cheese.

I had five consultant teams to look after my case. They were the consultant in Obstetrics & Gynaecology, Consultant in Fetal Medicine & Obstetrics, Consultant in Maternal Medicine & Obstetrics, A specialist registrar to the Perinatal Clinic and the renal consultant team. They set up a joint clinic between antenatal and renal clinic. I had been booked for uterine artery Dopplers when my gestation at 24 weeks.

A couple weeks before I was at 13 weeks gestation, I had attended the renal clinic, my renal function has been reasonably stable and I was having regular follow up with the renal team at Addenbrooke, my test results were Haemoglobin 11.7; urea 6.8; Creatinine 92; GFR 63, blood pressure 128/90 and my urine was negative. I was on Tacrolimus, Azathioprine, Folic acid and Prednisolone.

# At Perinatal Clinic

The specialist registrar had discussed the particular risks of declining renal function and

Hypertension/Pre-Eclampsia developments in the pregnancy with me. I was also aware of the risks of fetal growth retardation.

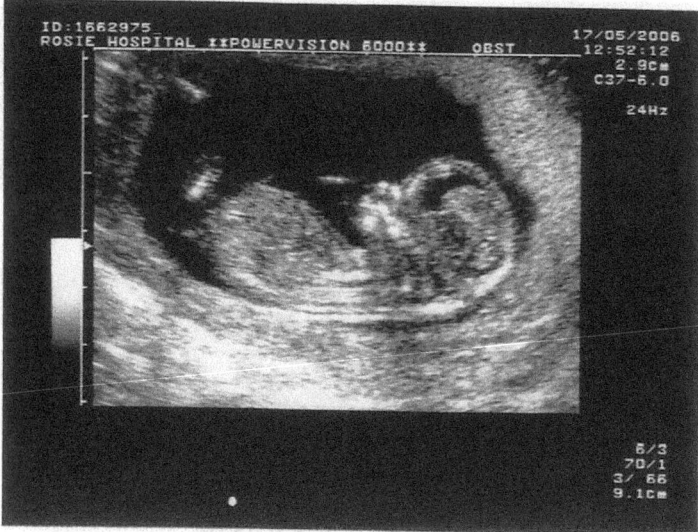

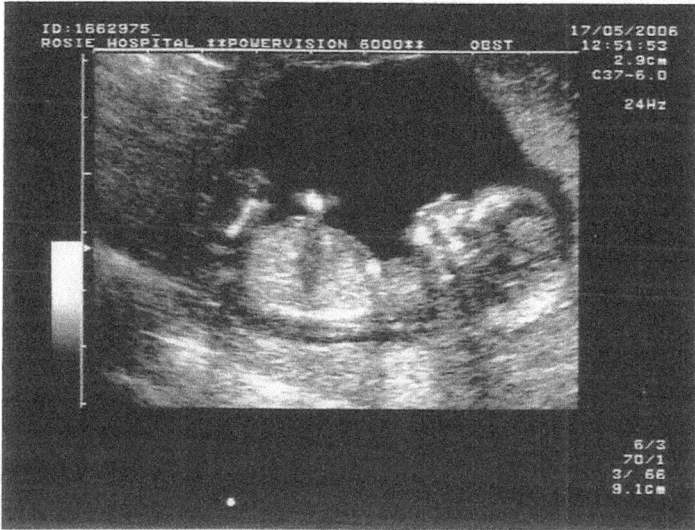

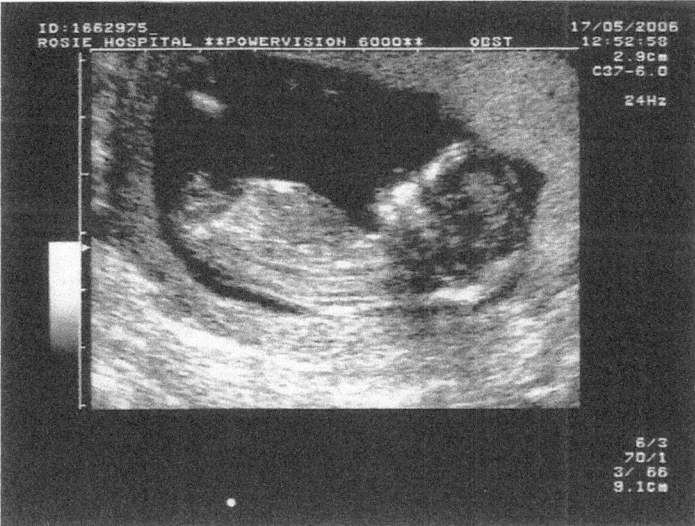

Dr. Kesorn Pechrach Weaver                    23

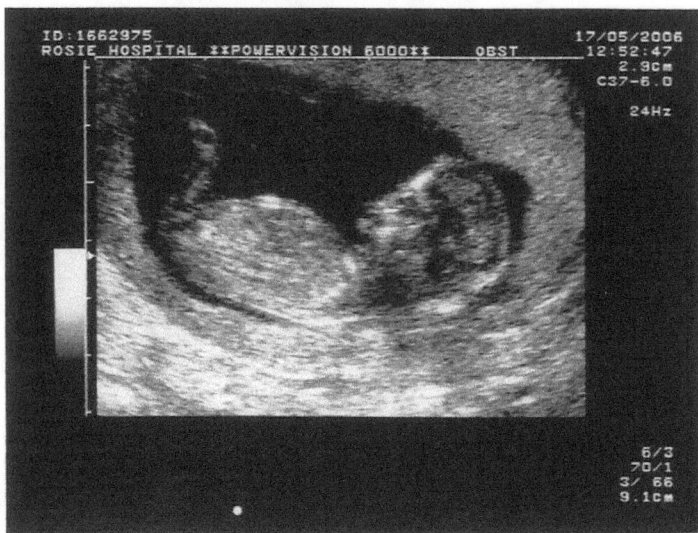

Figure 3.1: First scan at 12 weeks

# 16 Weeks

I have no further appointed with the Rosie hospital until the next scan of 20 weeks. However, we do pay for a private for Down syndrome scanner. This is a special scan to check the amount of water before the neck of his fetus when its age about 16 weeks. My husband and I agree that if it is high risk to be Down syndrome from the scan results. We will go for termination because we do not want our baby grow up as the condition. Not be born is better than in the condition. Anyway, the results

come out just fine, low risk. One more tests have
been passed.

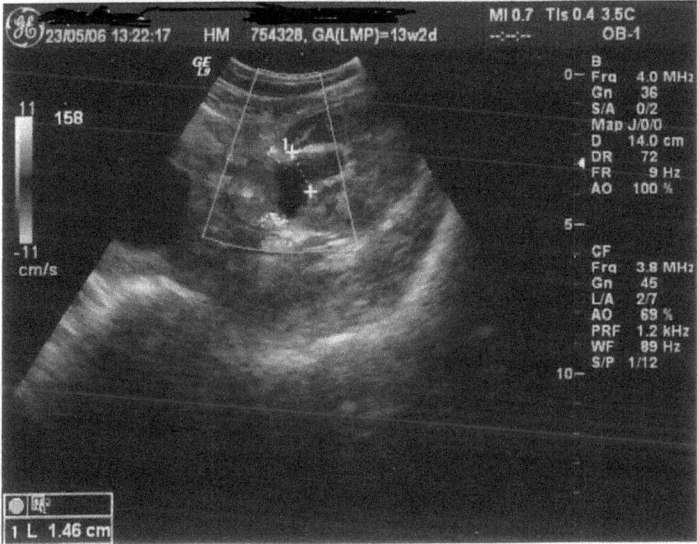

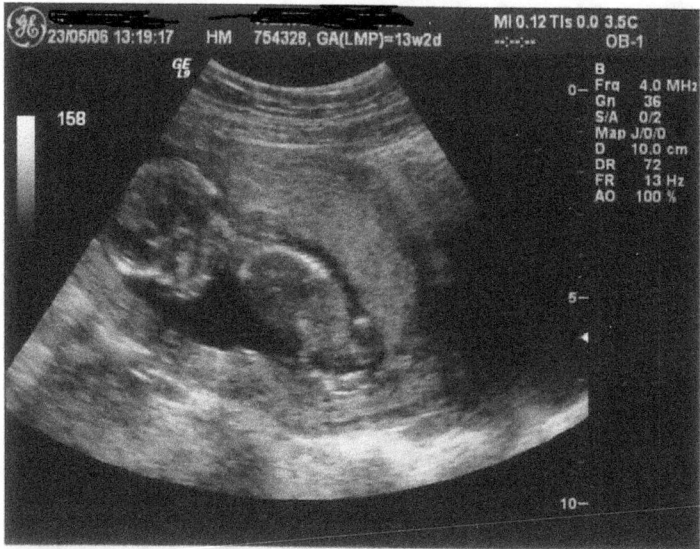

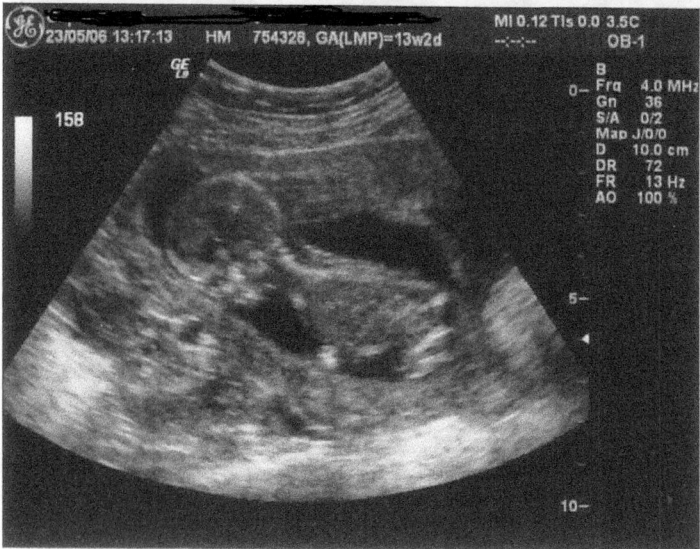

Born from Kidney Transplant Mother

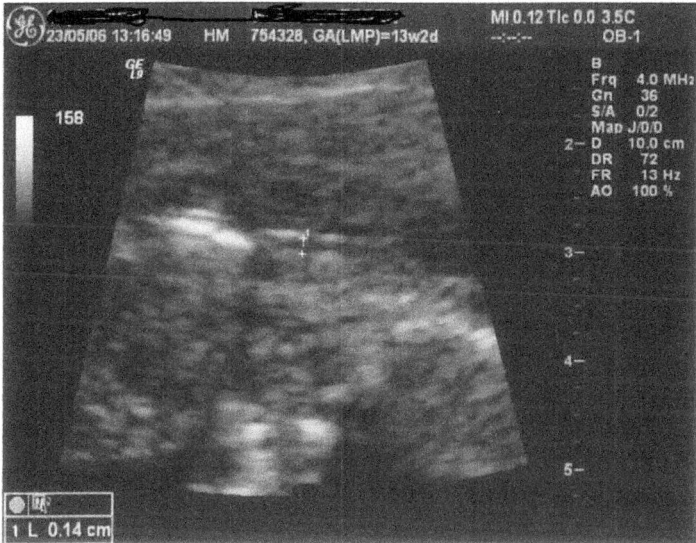

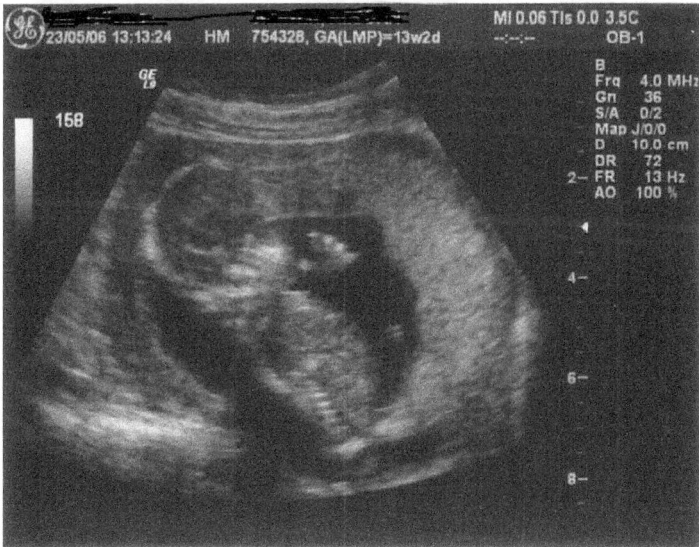

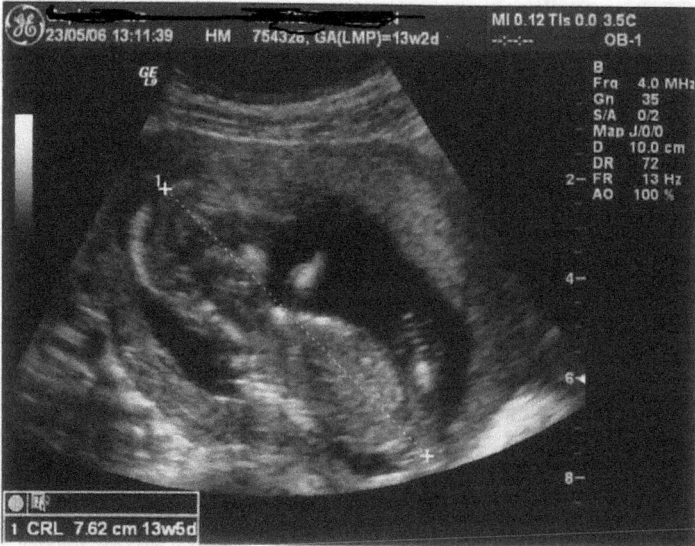

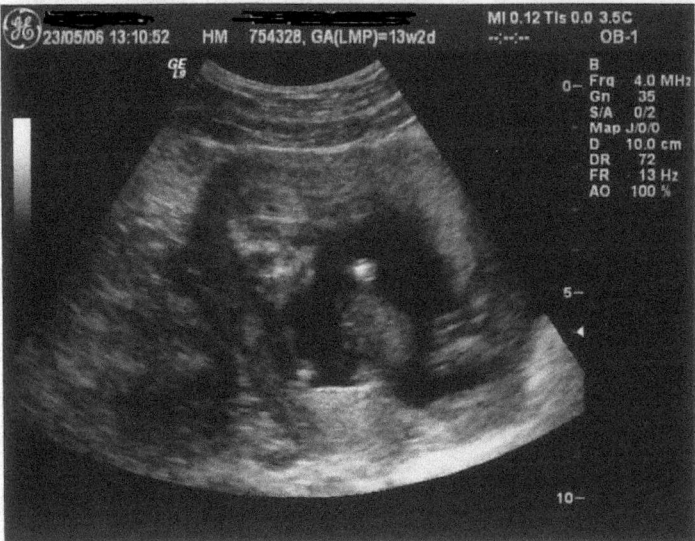

Figure 3.2: Private scans for checking Down

Born from Kidney Transplant Mother

I feel more relaxed and live a normal life. I work, do housework, cleaning, shopping and regular swimming which is the only sport that they said it is good for pregnant woman. Also, I do walk more and I enjoy it.

# 20 Weeks

Week by week pass easily and my tummy starts to show off a little bit. This may be because my build is a small and slender shape. It is easy to notice the node, stick out from the middle of my body.

I have an appointment with the ultrasound scangrapher. With the further development of the baby size, they can find out the sex of the baby inside. She does some checking of the size of the head and the size of the stomach and tells us the baby is in the right size for the age. Everything is fine and she makes us another scan appoint at the next 4 weeks. We come home to the delight because we know that we are going to have a boy.

My husband prepares a new room for a baby and I start to look at the baby catalogue for furniture, clothes, cot, bed, etc. We went shopping to look at the buggy technology in the shopping more and I eat more amount of food and more often than before. I also thought I had to eat for two. Also, I am regularly swim, the exercise is still on the same schedule.

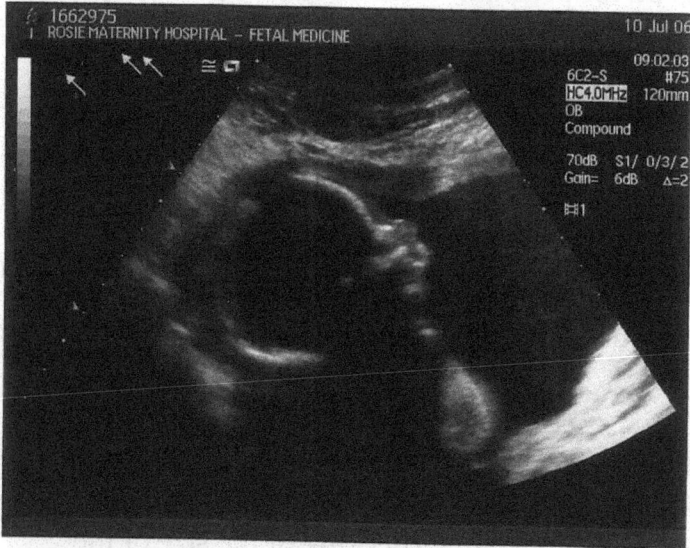

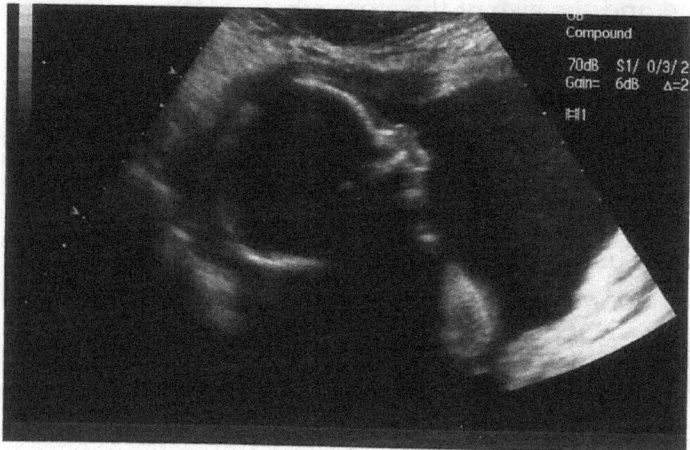

Born from Kidney Transplant Mother

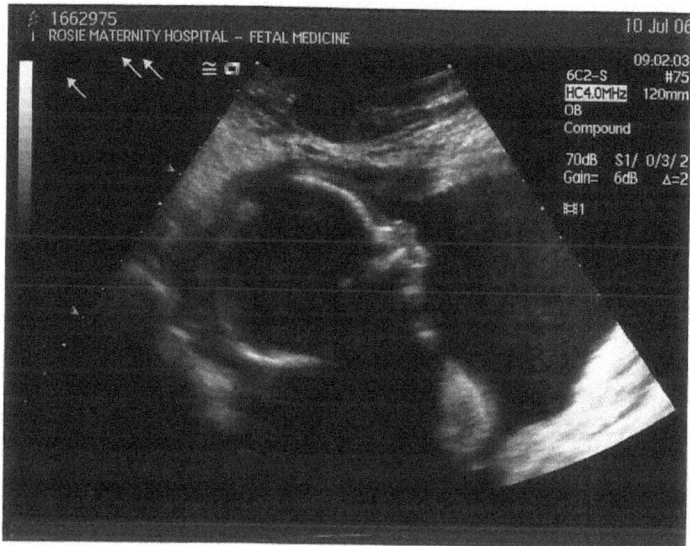

Figure 3.3: Scan at 20 weeks

# 23 Weeks and 5 days

This is another appointment for the ultrasound
scans. I did not feel so much exciting this time
since I have come here a few times, get to the know
the place, get the know people, know where to
park the car, which routes to walk in the hospital.
The process is the same, arrive at the reception
desk, she acknowledges that we have arrived; go to
the siting areas and waiting for the appointment
time. I have never been late for my appointment, I
am always being early. However, the clinic has

rarely run on time anyway. If I was late and the schedule is on time, I will miss my appointment, which they have to do that to be fair to other people. I cannot blame them because every slot is fixed by the time. If I am on time for my slot, although the clinic is late. The staff will work longer hour until the whole waiting areas are empty.

My appointment today is in the mid afternoon, few people after us. This time we see a woman as scanner officer. She has been checking for a while to measure the head and the tommy size of the baby. After that, she checks the flow spikes of the blood flow in and flow out in the placenta areas. She asked me to wait for a while before she lefts the room and come back with a man. He introduced himself to me as a specialist. He sits instead of the woman's position and starts to scan my tummy again. I can sense that there must have something is not right. This is like the second opinion. It does not take long before he wipes all of gel out of my tummy and asks my husband and me to meet with specialist teams. They will explain the results to me.

While we are waiting in the silent room, I can feel the steady of the air around me, I look at my husband. He keeps his face very well, did not show any signs at all. The pediatrician comes to us with all of the scan results data. She starts to explain to us that the baby stopped growing since 20 weeks. During last 3-4 weeks, the baby has been starving because of the flow resistance between the mother and the baby side is high. This result in the head of the baby still keeps growing while the tummy size is reduced. This should be opposite because the tummy is the source of food to feed the brain and growth other parts of the body. However, when the baby is in the situation of not a lot of food left, they baby needs to keep the brain growth but reduce the activity in somewhere else.

This time there is not much option to choose because the baby is less than 24 weeks. The outcome was very poor. She explained to us there is only a Caesarian section to take the baby out when he was 24 weeks. Due to the baby is very young in age; some body parts were not completely developed. There is a chance that the baby can be blind, deaf, low IQ caused by the early brain development and he may be not able to walk. However, this is the possibility of the medical research and the doctors' experience.

What they have to do now is admitted me in the hospital for a couple days until the baby is fully at 24 weeks. They allow my husband to stay overnight with me in the individual room. The nurse connects me to the heart monitor to check the baby's heartbeat. The night has gone by slowly, the nurse come to my room to check the blood pressure and normal routine check.

Morning on Thursday I remember everything clearly it does not matter how long it has passed. When people said time heal, I agree, but I always remember and I will remember for how long I do not know. The male comes in saying good morning and put the heart monitor around my tummy as usual. This time is quiet, so sound, no signal. He said the machine may have some problem. He goes and fetches a new one. I know it with my sense that the baby was gone since last night. This time I accept the real situation easily than the previous one when I had my miscarriage at 3 months. However, the new machine confirms the worst and it is my first time I see the tear from my husband's eyes.

I run out of words, nothing to say about it. We do everything that they told us to do. Again, I go into the induce process. I ask them why they will not perform a Caesarian Section. They said it is not necessary because the baby is dead. There is no need to be hurry and it will put straight in my body after the operation. The best is just do normal give birth via virginal. They give me morphine and I have a button to control myself. They suggest do not let my body feel painful.

After breakfast they give me tablets to start the procedure. Most of the time I just lay down in my bed and my husband always is by my side. They inserted some tablets inside my virginity in the afternoon to speed up the induce process. I started to feel something moving inside me about 7-8 PM in the night. Suddenly, I have an urge to go to the toilet. I can feel like some lower part of my body is going to drop off. My husband and a midwife carry me side by side go to the toilet. Just in time there is a big gust of some big thing was dropped inside the toilet. I think it must be my baby drop out. Anyway, it is not, the midwife explains to me that that is the water break.

Mid of the night, I do not know anything; I press my morphine any time I feel pain. I half sleep and half awake. I see the room is very dark, all curtains are black. There is only one headlight on. I see only two people, one is my husband and another one is the midwife who she comes to check me from time to time to see how big its open. I drill in and drill off half dream, half sleep, half awake and I just feel tired and want to sleep and want to have this bad dream finished.

The midwife comes in and this time she asks me to push. She explains to me like to push like go to the toilet. I did as she told me a few times and she told me the baby was out. I have no ideas and any feeling at all the baby come out and I just want to go back to my sleep. I remember she asked if I want to see and hold the baby. I said no and I went back to sleep again. I feel the sharp snap in the leg, the midwife just injects me. She explains to me this medicine is for the placenta and the remaining which have to come out. If not, they still connect to my womb and I will lose my blood from them. This time I can feel something like sleepily come out and I hear the midwife counting something. She explains to me that all of the placenta roots have to come out. If there is some remaining, she has to perform and use a dilator and removing any remaining tissue with a suction device.

Friday morning, I did not feel like I have slept at all. I feel like I have a long night travel in the straight place meet and see a lot of things and many things happen. The curtain was drawn. I just see it is not a dark black room anymore. I asked my husband if it is the same room as the last night of they move me after giving birth finish. He confirms I have been in the same room all night until the morning. I still feel extremely tired and want to go back to sleep, I do not want to wash or have any breakfast. However, the nurse does not allow me to do that. I have been washed, feed breakfast; all of the tubes were coming out of my hand. My tummy is still big and I have to wear the sanitary in my underwear.

The same nurse to us with a big paper and document. I ask my husband to due to them since my brain was not completely function. I still feel half awake and half sleepy. However, I still can hear some questions she asks us about if we want to know the results of the baby examination, do we want to have the baby funeral or we want them to do it and much more. She always said that she wants us to leave within today because it is Friday, if not we have to stay for the weekend and have to leave on Monday. Therefore, we have to sign all of documents quickly and she gives us the counselor's telephone number in case we may need it later. That is all and we are in the car on Friday daytime, I still half sleep and half awake. When we get home, I went to have a lay down on the sofa while my husband goes to do gardening in the back of our house.

# Post Mortem

I had been given the booklet of the consent to a hospital post mortem examination on a baby. We called him baby Weaver because we had not thought about his name to be yet and also this happens so suddenly. This agreement, consent has six sections and it was quite easy to follow. It likes questionnaires.

- Agreement to full post mortem examination.
- Limiting the post mortem examination.
- Agree to donation of tissue and fluid samples for use in medical research.
- Genetic testing
- Consent for retention of whole organs and tissue (other than blocks and slides), their uses and options for disposal.

  o Consent for retention of organs and tissue for more detailed examination.

  o Donation of organs for medical research, education or audit.

- Disposal of retained organs and tissue.

Born from Kidney Transplant Mother

# Chapter 4

# 3rd Pregnancy: Premature

This pregnancy is my third time, I would say to get pregnant is not difficult for me, but to keep it going is not successful yet. My husband and I have some discussion and this will be the last pregnancy. If thing has gone wrong, we will stop and just to accept our family is only two of us.

With the experience to two lots at 12 weeks and 24 weeks. I consider myself as professional pregnancies that pass them all. I learn a lot of miscarriage and stillbirth. I read a lot of books do a lot of research in journals and update all of medical journal papers and conference about pregnancy. I should get another Ph.D. in pregnant woman.

However, the previous till birth, the doctors could not count as general case any more. It is not 80% will happen to them as they reference to miscarriage case. They said they will investigate and see what happen why the blood flow stops or have resistance to the baby side after 20 weeks pregnancy.

We have an appointment to listen to the test results from the paediatrician. They found nothing wrong with the baby side while the renal consultant teams confirm everything in their response is completely correct. They have been changing my medicine about 6 months before I started to get the first pregnancy. They confirm all of my anti-rejection medicine or post kidney transplant medicine have been changed to the safety dose. The effect of this medication would not affect t the pregnancy at all. Anyway, nobody faults that I lost my baby this second time. We call it "the act of god".

Getting pregnant is not different from other woman. However, with transplant woman may be a little bit harder than others. This is because of suppressive medicines to prevent organ rejection.

The process to see the doctors may be more frequent than normal, healthy woman, but that to make sure everything is to manage.

At least this is proof that transplant woman can have a baby just like the other woman. We as transplant lady we can have our baby.

# 4 Weeks

After self pregnancy test at home for couple times, it is time to inform the GP. This is the starting point; the GP will inform the renal consultants, Obstetrician, neonatal consultants, Paediatrician, local midwife and Health visitor. You can see it is not only a doctor or a midwife, but it is teams of specialist to look after each case.

# 8 Weeks

Live a normal life, eat and sleep the same pattern as usual. It may feel a little bit tired and hungry more often. However, this is normal just like other women do while they are pregnant. The GP may ask to come in for blood pressure and general check.

# 9 Weeks

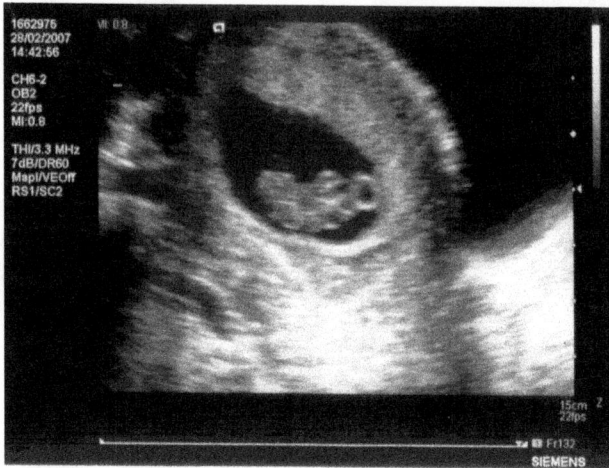

**Examination**

Time 14:56

Department: Obstetric Ultrasound Dept, Rosie

**Ultrasound**

US system Siemens Antares
transabdominal

Gestational age 8 weeks + 5 days

EDD by scan 05/10/07

**First Trimester Ultrasound**

Findings normal intrauterine pregnancy

Fetal heart activity present

CRL 22.0 mm |——•——|

Amniotic fluid normal

Thank you for referring your patient

Ultrasound demonstrated a singleton pregnancy compatible with 8 weeks and 5 days. Incidental note is made of a 24mm corpus luteum originating from the right ovary. The left ovary is not positively identified. 11-14 and 20 week scan booked.

Figure 4.1: Scan at 9 weeks

# 12 Weeks

The first semester I have no excitement anymore. I prepare to accept any news good and bad. Although it is good now and it can always go bad later. Therefore, every minute is changeable. The best for me just live day by day, no hope no plan. "When it is there, it's there". If it does not mean to be, that is alright for me.

I inform my GP as usual after the first four weeks when I do my pregnancy test and see the two blue lines. Again he gives me folic acid and this time he does not need to tell me anything. I know best what will happen and what to do with it.

When I went to see my renal consultant, they request to see me as soon as I get pregnant. This time they give Aspirin add to my kidney transplant medication. They told me Aspirin can help to thin my blood. I understand when the blood is thinner, it can flow passes the filter in placenta between mother and baby side easily than before. Well, I do anything that I have been told.

After seeing the GP as usual, this is the first critical point, this is the first ultrasound by the Ultra sonographer to see the viability of the fetus. It means to check if there is a heart beat inside the womb.

"If there is one, congratulation! You have it".

Although the picture of the scan, print out see something like a small bean shape. That is why we always call our baby "The bean".

If there is "not", it may be hard to accept it. It is a bad news. It does not matter what other people try to say anything, such as it happens to normal, healthy woman too, or it has not just developed to be, etc. As a transplant woman always thinks it is because of the drugs I have to take it every day.

From my history of miscarriage and stillbirth, the renal consultants add aspirin in my medicine collection. This is believed to help the flow of my blood pass placenta better.

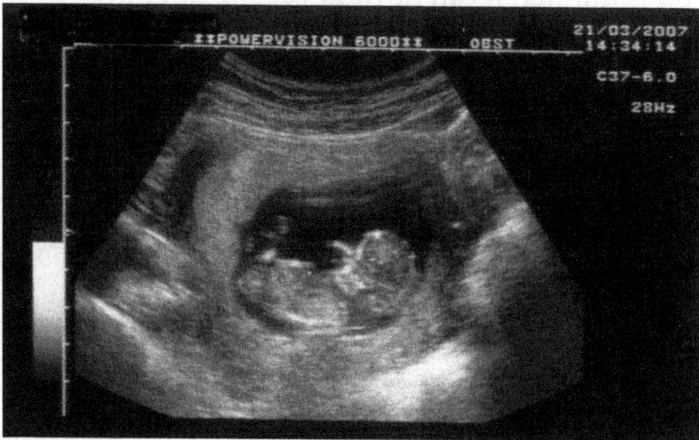

**Ultrasound**

US system   Toshiba Powervision
transabdominal

View   good

Gestational age   11 weeks + 5 days

EDD by scan   05/10/07

**First Trimester Ultrasound**

Findings   normal intrauterine pregnancy

Fetal heart activity   present

CRL   49.7  mm        ⊢——⊕——⊣

Thank you for referring your patient
Ultrasound demonstrated a singleton pregnancy compatible with 11 weeks and 5 days.
Previously noted corpus luteal type of cyst within the right ovary now measures 19.8 x 15.4 x 19mm.
The left ovary appears normal. LIF transplanted kidney is noted.
20 weeks scan has been booked.

Figure 4.2: Scan at 12 weeks

# Scan 12 Weeks and 1 day

EDD: 05 October 2007, EDD by dates: 05 October 2007

**First Trimester Ultrasound:**                                        Examination date: 24 March 2007
US machine: GE Logic9. Probe: C4 - 2. Visualisation: good.
**Gestational age: 12 weeks + 1 days** from dates                      EDD by scan: 05 October 2007
Findings:                         normal intrauterine pregnancy
Fetal heart activity present.
Crown-rump length (CRL)                                57.8 mm      |——•——|
Biparietal diameter (BPD)                              20.0 mm
Nuchal translucency (NT)                               1.1 mm
Placenta:                                              anterior low
Amniotic fluid:                                        normal
Cord:                                                  not examined
**Fetal anatomy:**
**Skull/brain:** appears normal; **Spine:** appears normal; **Abdomen:** appears normal; **Stomach:** visible; **Bladder:** not visible; **Hands:** both visible; **Feet:** both visible;
**Comments:** A small right sided ovarian cyst is noted measuring 1.8 x 1.7 cm in size.
Transplanted mothers kidney noted in left side of pelvis.

**Comments**
The patient will discuss the findings with her midwife / Consultant.

The Nuchal translucency has reduced the age related risk for chromosomal abnormalities. A routine 19 - 22 week scan should be performed to rule out structural defects.
**Estimated risk for Trisomy 21 (Down's syndrome), 18 (Edward's syndrome) + 13 (Patau's syndrome):**
Patient counselled and consent given
Maternal age:                                          38 years
Background risk of Trisomy 21                          1: 131
Adjusted risk of Trisomy 21                            **1: 704**
Background risk of Trisomy 13+18                        1: 233
Adjusted risk of Trisomy 13+18                         **1: 2187**

*The background risk is based on maternal age. The adjusted risk is the risk at the time of screening, calculated on the basis of the background risk and ultrasound factors (fetal nuchal translucency thickness)*
*The model for adjustment of risk is based on findings from more than 100,000 patients who have participated in research coordinated by the Fetal Medicine Foundation, (Registered charity 1037116). The risk is only valid if the NT measurement was performed by a sonographer who has been accredited by the Fetal Medicine Foundation (see www.fetalmedicine.com).*

## First Trimester Screening Report

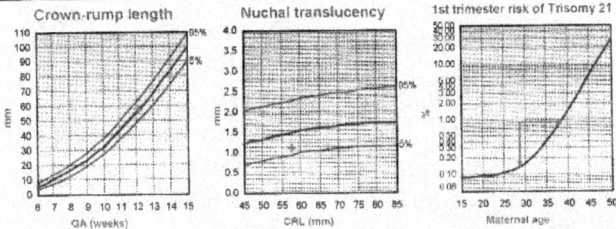

Crown-rump length     Nuchal translucency     1st trimester risk of Trisomy 21

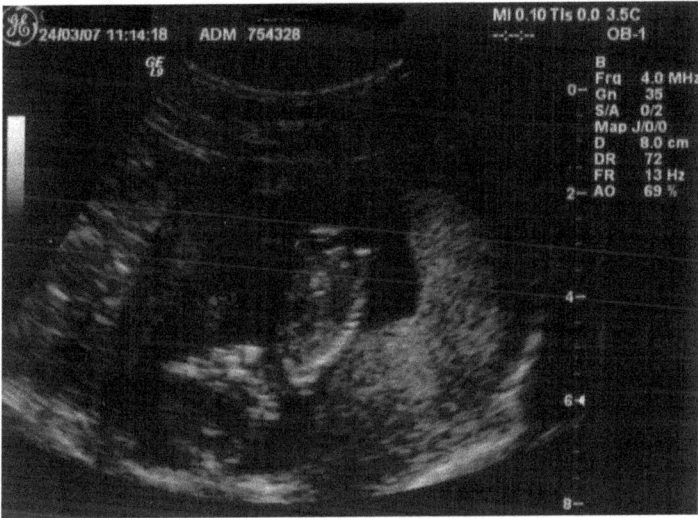

Figure 4.3: Scan for checking Down syndrome

The third pregnancy, we have solid plan more than the previous two pregnancies. My plan is no plan, live day by day. I just realise people who have nothing to think about, nothing to worry, nothing at all, how they feel. It is empty, out of control. It does not mater how good I did, how brilliant I prepare, it does not guarantee the results at all. It is not as simple as a formula in engineering rule or mathematic law.

The GP asks to check my blood pressure in the surgery every other day. I will be seen in the renal clinic every other week similar to the pediatrician to see every other week. The scan clinic will see me every two weeks. Therefore, my routine will visit a clinic in the hospital one a week between pediatrician clinic and renal clinic. Some weeks I have two clinics attend in one day. The good thing is all the clinics are in the same areas, but they operate in the different day.

# 14 Weeks

I know earlier that this time at 12 weeks I will have Asplirin as well as continue on folic acid from previous months.

I go for the routine scan to check the visibility of the heart beat. This is the starting point for the pregnancy progress. I feel nothing and a bit happy to hear the baby's heartbeat. However, from my previous experience of the lost at 24 weeks, that pregnancy is still in my mind. It is never easy for me to get maximum happiness as before. I always put the break at 50% in the case of the worst thing happen; I will not hurt too much. As well as starting to take aspirin and folic, I still take all kidney transplant medicine to suppress my immunity system

I was wondering really why it also counts in week, but that is how it works. If the counts in the day, it may not easy to see how different the fetus grows. Blood pressure check with a GP is still the routine check.

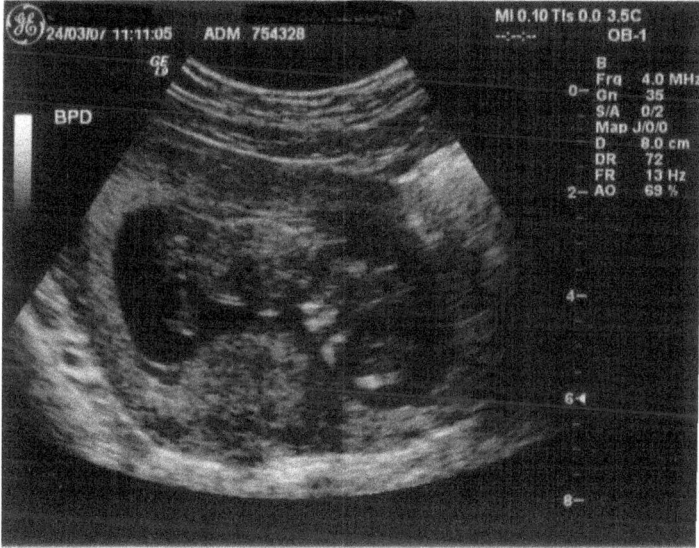

Figure 4.4: Scan for Spinal Bifida

I am sure you will be pleased to hear that your recent maternal screening test has shown that your baby is not at high risk for Down syndrome or Spina Bifida.

We have combined the results of your triple test with the results of your nuchal scan to calculate the chance of Down syndrome in your pregnancy.

The results show that your chance of having a baby with Down syndrome is:

**1 : 348**

Out of every **348** women with the same result as you, **one** will have a baby with Down syndrome, and **347** will have unaffected babies.

A copy of this result has been sent to your family doctor and your hospital antenatal clinic.

If you have any questions about your result please do not hesitate to contact either your midwife

We wish you a very happy outcome to your pregnancy.

# Scan 16 Weeks and 3 days

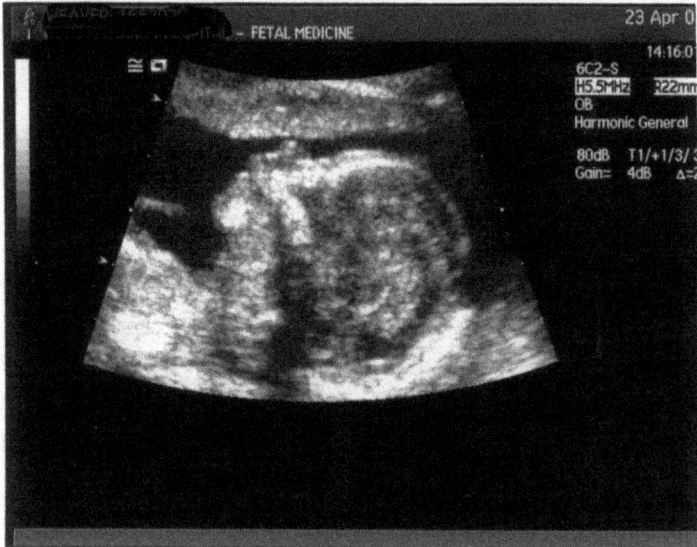

| US system | Acuson Sequoia |
| --- | --- |
| | transabdominal |
| View | good |
| Gestational age | 16 weeks + 3 days |
| EDD by scan | 05/10/07 |

**Biometry / Anatomy**

| | | |
| --- | --- | --- |
| BPD | 35.0 mm | ⊢——▸——⊣ |
| HC | 126.0 mm | ⊢—•—⊣ |
| AC | 107.0 mm | ⊢ ·•· ·⊣ |
| FL | 21.0 mm | ⊢—•—⊣ |
| HC/AC | 1.18 | ⊢—•—⊣ |
| Fetal heart activity | present | |

| | |
| --- | --- |
| **Head** | normal skull shape |
| **Brain** | hemispheres, ventricles mid-brain and posterior fossa appear normal |
| **Face** | no facial cleft and the eyes, nose and mandible appear normal |
| **Spine** | no spina bifida or kyphoscoliosis |
| **Neck/Skin** | no skin oedema or cystic hygroma |
| **Thorax** | thorax and lungs appear normal |
| **Heart** | normal 4-chamber view |
| | (the great arteries were also examined and appear normal) |
| **Abdominal Wall** | no abdominal wall defect |
| **GIT** | stomach and GIT appear normal |
| **Urinary tract** | kidneys and bladder appear normal |
| **Extremities** | hands, feet, arms, legs and joints appear normal |
| **Genitalia** | normal genitalia (parents do not want to know sex) |

This patient attended for an early scan in view of a previous loss at 23+6. All views of the fetus were normal today. She will have a further anomaly scan at 20 weeks and uterine artery Doppler at 23 weeks. Further fetal assessment will be arranged following the 23 week scan.

Figure 4.5: Scan at 16 weeks

# Scan 16 weeks and 6 days

The routine to see the GP every week to check blood pressure is going well. Although we have a blood pressure machine at home, I still have to go to the surgery for blood pressure checking. The value of my blood pressure between the machine at home and the one in surgery is not the same but not far off. We can plot graphs and figures.

As always I went to private Down syndrome scan in the private hospital to check the liquid behind the neck of the fetus.

The renal consultant asked me to start my medication Tacrolimus 4 mg twice a day.

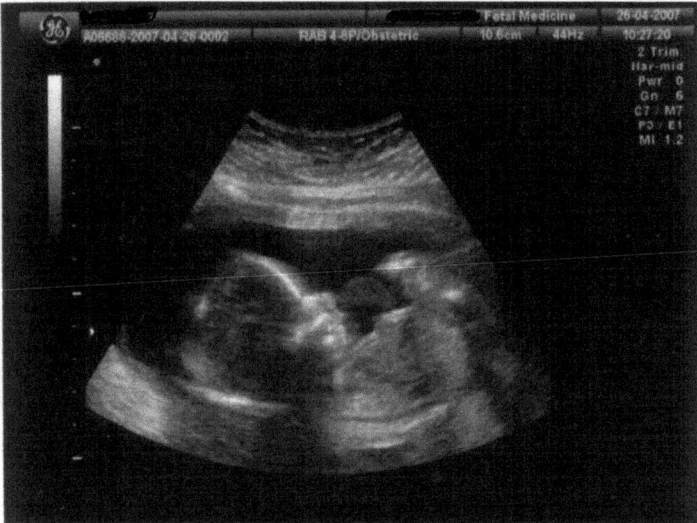

**Examination**

Time 10.18

Department Fetal Medicine Unit

**Ultrasound**

Operator

FMF operator code 24,533

US system Kretz Voluson 730

transabdominal

View good

Gestational age 16 weeks + 6 days

EDD by scan 05/10/07

**Biometry / Anatomy**

Fetal heart activity present

Fetal movements normal

Presentation breech

Amniotic fluid normal

**Doppler ultrasound**

**Uterine artery**

PI left 1.33

PI right 1.44

Mean PI 1.38

Notch **bilateral notch**

Assessment normal placental bloodflow

**Conclusions**

Diagnosis normal findings

**Renal transplant**
**Previous IUD: IUGR/PET at 23 weeks**

Left sided kidney. Scan earlier this week showed normal fetal growth.

Scan today shows normal uterine artery Doppler resistance, with small bilateral notches (notches are quite common at this gestation and do not have a sinister significance in the context of normal resistance). These findings are reassuring in that there is no obvious utero-placental problem, and the likelihood of early onset pre-eclampsia/fetal growth restriction occurring is low.

A 20 week scan is booked, and we will see back in fetal medicine at around 22/23 weeks.

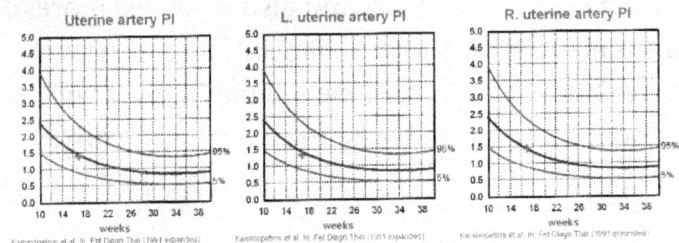

Figure 4.6: Doppler ultrasound to check the flow

# 19 Weeks

I have a Varicella Zoster immunity VZV IgG (Immunity), my antibody is positive an evidence of immunity to chickenpox.

# 20 Weeks

Here is the mid point or half way to pregnancy for normal woman, but not for us, transplant woman like us. It starts the critical points which have to look closely. Another routine scan will check the growth rate and can tell the sex of the fetus if we want to know. The Radiologist will check the blood flow in and flow out in the placenta, which this is the point that mother body supply food to her baby and collect all of waste back to her body.

It is an important period of pregnancy for transplant woman's body because the baby grows bigger, it needs more food and also it creates more waste out. With only one transplant kidney, now it is not only the waste from the woman herself only, but also plus addition waste from the baby grows inside her womb.

As I mention before, a kidney can train to work harder, but it must not to overload. When that time, there always show some signal such as blood pressure, chemicals in our blood from the blood test, the Creatinine level may be sky high going up within a short period.

The result of my blood test for Haemoglobin (Hb) is 10.1 g/dl. The normal range for a woman at the beginning of her pregnancy is 11.0 g/dl and above. During the course of pregnancy, the anticipate would fall slightly and by 28 weeks of pregnancy a Hb of 10.5 g/dl and above is considered to be within normal limits.

I have a new medication added to my lists; it is Ferrous Fumarate BP 210 mg (approximate 65 mg Ferrors irons). I have to take it twice a day. I still continue to take Folic acid because the folic acid will help my body to absorb the iron more efficiently.

# 20 Weeks and 3 days

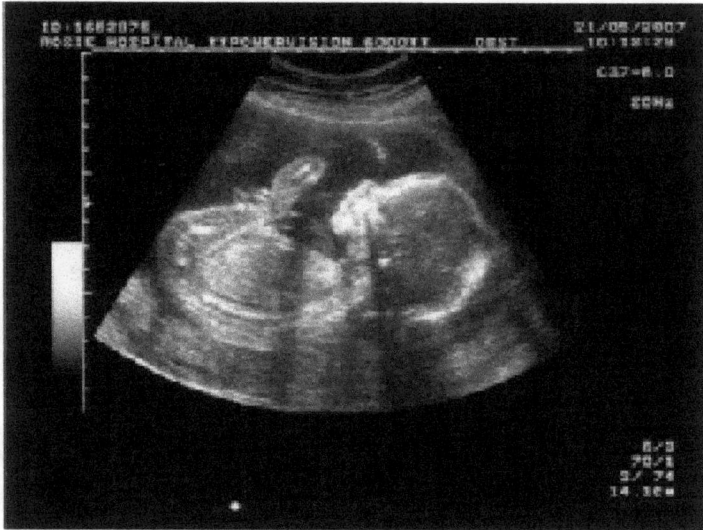

**Ultrasound**

Department Obstetric Ultrasound Dept. Rosie

Operator

US system Toshiba Powervision
transabdominal

View good

Gestational age 20 weeks + 3 days

EDD by scan 05/10/07

**Biometry / Anatomy**

| | | |
|---|---|---|
| BPD | 46.0 mm | |
| HC | 177.0 mm | |
| TCD | 20.2 mm | |
| AC | 157.3 mm | |
| FL | 33.5 mm | |
| HC/AC | 1.13 | |

Fetal heart activity present

Fetal movements normal

Placenta site anterior high

Amniotic fluid normal

Cord 3 vessels

**Head**            normal skull shape

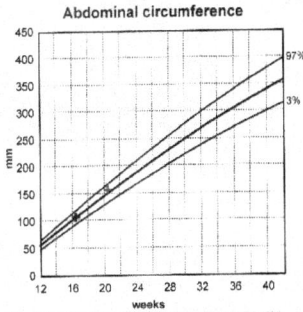
Abdominal circumference

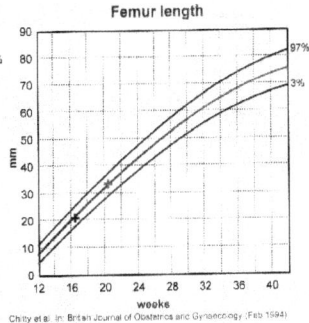
Femur length

Chitty et al. In: British Journal of Obstetrics and Gynaecology (Feb 1994)

| | |
|---|---|
| **Brain** | hemispheres, ventricles mid-brain and posterior fossa appear normal |
| **Face** | no facial cleft and the eyes, nose and mandibis appear normal |
| **Spine** | no spina bifida or kyphoscoliosis |
| **Neck/Skin** | no skin oedema or cystic hygroma |
| **Thorax** | thorax and lungs appear normal |
| **Heart** | normal 4-chamber view |
| | (the great arteries were also examined and appear normal) |
| **Abdominal Wall** | no abdominal wall defect |
| **GIT** | stomach and GIT appear normal |
| **Urinary tract** | kidneys and bladder appear normal |
| **Extremities** | hands, feet, arms, legs and joints appear normal |

Thank you for referring your patient
Ultrasound examination revealed no obvious fetal anomalies. Normal growth. Normal amniotic fluid. Good fetal movements.

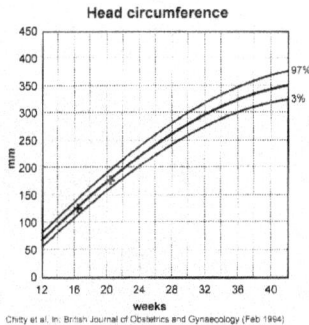
Head circumference

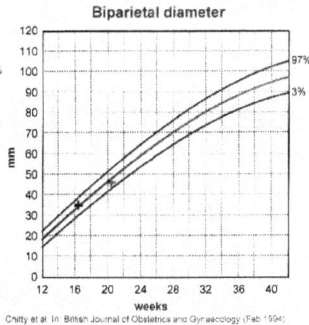
Biparietal diameter

Chitty et al. In: British Journal of Obstetrics and Gynaecology (Feb 1994)

Figure 4.7: Scan to check the growth

# 21 Weeks

The renal consultant asked me to adjust my medication Tacrolimus from 4 mg twice a day to 5 mg twice daily.

# 22 Weeks and 4 days

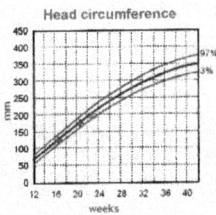

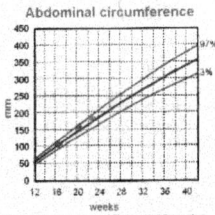

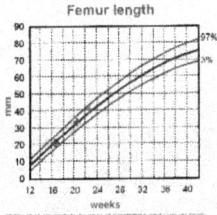

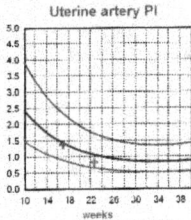

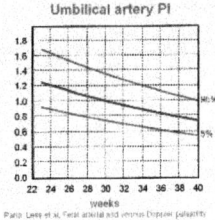

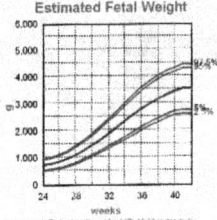

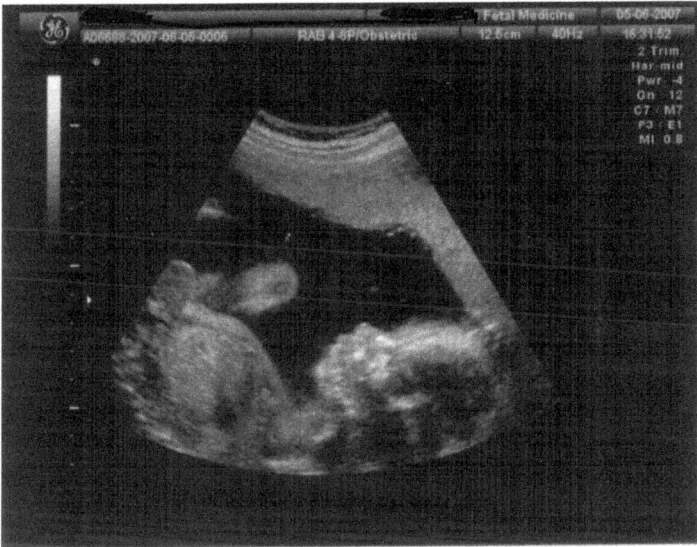

**Ultrasound**

Department Fetal Medicine Unit

Operator

FMF operator code 24,533

US system Kretz Voluson 730

transabdominal

View good

Gestational age 22 weeks + 4 days

EDD by scan 05/10/07

**Biometry / Anatomy**

BPD 53.8 mm

HC 195.7 mm

TCD 23.0 mm

AC 184.4 mm

FL 41.0 mm

HC/AC 1.06

Estimated fetal weight Hadlock (BPD-HC-AC-FL)

561 g

Fetal heart activity present

Fetal movements normal

Presentation cephalic

Placenta site anterior high

Amniotic fluid normal

**Doppler ultrasound**

Uterine artery

PI left 0.71

PI right 0.91

Mean PI 0.81

Notch no notch

Umbilical artery

PI 1.20

EDF positive

Assessment normal fetal and placental Doppler

**Conclusions**

Diagnosis normal findings

**Renal transplant (left sided kidney)**
**Previous IUD: IUGR/PET at 23 weeks**

Normal fetal growth, amniotic fluid and movements. Uterine artery Doppler is normal with no notches indicating a reassuringly low risk of early onset fetal growth restriction or pre-eclampsia. Umbilical artery Doppler is also normal.

Fortunately, Kesum's blood pressure is well controlled; it is being checked weekly at present. We will see her in clinic with a prior scan in 3 weeks, and 2 weekly scans/perinatal clinic appointments thereafter.

Figure 4.8: Doppler ultrasound at 22 weeks

Born from Kidney Transplant Mother

# 24 Weeks

This is the starting point of the baby able to survive. It means that when the fetus reach at this age, it can be born survive, but it may develop disable such as deaf, blind, and other disable. This is because the brain other organs have not developed properly.

Once again, the Radiologist will check blood flow in and out in the placenta areas. The ultrasound and scan by Ultrasonographer will perform to measure the head and stomach size of the baby sees the how the baby grows inside the body.

I have been given Labetalol to lower my blood pressure, 100 mg twice a day. Blood pressure check with GP performs 2-3 times a week to check and catch the blood pressure rise. This can lead to Pre-Eclampsia which is a pregnancy complication characterized by high blood pressure and signs of damage to another organ system.

# 26 Weeks

The Physiotherapy in outpatients department Herts & Essex Hospital has arranged an appointment for fembrace. I have been issued with number 3 fembrace to support the pelvis during pregnancy whilst the ligaments are lax.

My blood test for Haemoglobin (Hb) is 10.2 g/dl, which is lower than normal pregnancy at 11.0 fg/dl. It is also lower than the 28 weeks of pregnancy Hb of 10.5 g/dl.

# 27 Weeks

The renal consultant asked me to adjust my medication Tacrolimus from 5 mg twice a day to 6 mg twice daily.

At this point all of my doctor's team is pretty happy with my pregnancy progress. They start to get me in Steroid by dripping and medicine. This steroid will help to develop the lung system in the baby in case they have to get it out emergency which can happen anytime from now if my blood pressure going up and they cannot control it and bring it down to the safe level.

The ultrasound scan may perform or may be not, but there is new equipment adding at this stage. It is the machine to listen to the baby's heartbeat to check if it is in the stress condition.

The renal consultant asked me to adjust my medication Tacrolimus from 6 mg twice a day to 4 mg twice daily.

# 28 Weeks

My Tacrolimus is 2.3 and Creatinine is 117, therefore, the renal consultant asked me to adjust my medication Tacrolimus from 4 mg twice a day to 5 mg twice daily.

# 30 Weeks

The Physiotherapy in outpatients department Herts & Essex Hospital has been issued me with number 4 fembrace to support the pelvis during pregnancy.

The renal consultant called to adapt my transplant renal medication, my Creatinine 109, Tacrolimus level 5.5. Thus, continue Tacrolimus at 5 mg twice a day.

# 31 Weeks

The renal consultant called to inform the Creatinine level 123, Tacrolimus 5.2. Thus, continue Tacrolimus at 5 mg twice a day.

I have been asked to adjust the medication Labetalol to 200 mg in the morning and 100mg in the night.

## 32 Weeks

The renal consultant change the 210 mg Ferrous Fumarate to Ferrous Sulphate 200 mg twice a day, also adjust the Labetalol to 200 mg twice a day.

My blood pressure has gone up and down since weeks 28, however, after increasing the dose of blood pressure to the maximum and also add every kind of blood pressure medicines; the blood pressure is still high. It is time for emergency C-section.

Of course, it means that there must have a cot for the new born baby in the neonatal unit, SCUBU unit.

The consultant in Fetal Medicine & Obstetrics asked to stop Folic acid and Aspirin one day after delivering. Three days after delivery, he asked to adjust the Labetalol to 100 mg twice a day. The renal consultant asked to stop Ferrous Fumerate after delivery 2 days.

Name

Number

## Size charts

The most helpful way to understand scan results is to plot them on these charts using the **agreed due date**. Most correctly plotted results in a healthy pregnancy should be within the shaded areas on the graph. A trend in results is more important than a single result. Taller and heavier mothers tend to have heavier babies; shorter, lighter mothers have lighter babies.

## Ultrasound scans

| Date | Gestation | CRL | BPD | FL |
|------|-----------|-----|-----|-----|
|  |  |  |  |  |
|  |  |  |  |  |
|  |  |  |  |  |
|  |  |  |  |  |

Baby's head circumference in millimetres

Baby's abdominal circumference in millimetres

Baby's femur length in millimetres

Weeks of pregnancy

Scans 14-15

⊙ is used if plotting by menstrual due date

⊗ by agreed due date if different

Crown rump length in millimetres

Weeks of pregnancy

Please use **black ink** to fill in this record (photocopy friendly)

©NMRP V2.1 8/99

## Table: 4.1: Size chart from ultrasound scans

| HC | AC | Liquor | Placenta | Presenting | Fetal Heart | Comments | Signature |
|----|----|--------|----------|------------|-------------|----------|-----------|
| | | | | | | | |
| | | | | | | | |
| | | | | | | | |
| | | | | | | | |
| | | | | | | | |
| | | | | | | | |
| | | | | | | | |
| | | | | | | | |
| | | | | Results written in space above or top of first report fixed here | | | |

**Crown rump length and Biparietal diameter dating tables**

This chart is to help your care provider to confirm your agreed due date (average weeks plus days for each millimetre of measurement.)

**(CRL) Crown rump length – baby's head to bottom**

| size | weeks | size | weeks | size | weeks | size | weeks |
|------|-------|------|-------|------|-------|------|-------|
| 4 | 6+0 | 26 | 9+3 | 48 | 11+4 | 70 | 13+2 |
| 6 | 6+3 | 28 | 9+5 | 50 | 11+5 | 72 | 13+3 |
| 8 | 6+6 | 30 | 9+6 | 52 | 11+6 | 74 | 13+4 |
| 10 | 7+2 | 32 | 10+1 | 54 | 12+1 | 76 | 13+5 |
| 12 | 7+4 | 34 | 10+2 | 56 | 12+2 | 78 | 13+6 |
| 14 | 7+6 | 36 | 10+4 | 58 | 12+3 | 80 | 14+0 |
| 16 | 8+2 | 38 | 10+5 | 60 | 12+4 | | |
| 18 | 8+3 | 40 | 10+6 | 62 | 12+5 | | |
| 20 | 8+5 | 42 | 11+0 | 64 | 12+6 | | |
| 22 | 9+0 | 44 | 11+2 | 66 | 13+0 | | |
| 24 | 9+2 | 46 | 11+3 | 68 | 13+1 | | |

**(BPD) Biparietal diameter – width of baby's head**

| size | weeks | size | weeks | size | weeks | size | weeks |
|------|-------|------|-------|------|-------|------|-------|
| 18 | 12+1 | 29 | 14+6 | 40 | 18+1 | 51 | 21+4 |
| 19 | 12+3 | 30 | 15+1 | 41 | 18+3 | 52 | 22+0 |
| 20 | 12+4 | 31 | 15+3 | 42 | 18+5 | 53 | 22+2 |
| 21 | 12+6 | 32 | 15+5 | 43 | 19+0 | 54 | 22+4 |
| 22 | 13+1 | 33 | 16+0 | 44 | 19+3 | 55 | 23+0 |
| 23 | 13+2 | 34 | 16+2 | 45 | 19+5 | 56 | 23+2 |
| 24 | 13+4 | 35 | 16+4 | 46 | 20+0 | 57 | 23+4 |
| 25 | 13+6 | 36 | 16+6 | 47 | 20+2 | 58 | 23+6 |
| 26 | 14+1 | 37 | 17+1 | 48 | 20+4 | 59 | 24+2 |
| 27 | 14+3 | 38 | 17+4 | 49 | 21+0 | 60 | 24+4 |
| 28 | 14+5 | 39 | 17+6 | 50 | 21+2 | | |

Scans 14-15

Crown rump length dating table after Robinson and Fleming. Br J Obstet Gynaecol 1975 Vol.82, pp.702-710.
Biparietal diameter dating table based on 'outer to inner' measurements after Chitty et al. Br J Obstet Gynaecol 1994 Vol.101, pp.35-13.
Scan size charts show 3rd, 50th and 97th centiles.
Head circumference (HC), curve formula fitted results based on 'derived' (two diameter elipse method) circumference after Chitty et al. Br J Obstet Gynaecol 1994 Vol.101, pp.35-43.
Abdominal circumference (AC), curve formula fitted results based on 'derived' (two diameter elipse method) circumference after Chitty et al. Br J Obstet Gynaecol 1994 Vol.101, pp.125-131.
Femur length (FL), curve formula fitted results after Chitty et al. Br J Obstet Gynaecol 1994 Vol.101, pp.132-135.

# Table 4.2: Crown rump length and Biparietal diameter

# Chapter 5

# Giving Birth

It is normal procedure and high risk like me. Thus, I had to test for Hyperglycaemia with a non-fasting Lucozade challenge test during pregnancy at approximate 28 weeks gestation. If the results are above a certain threshold, then the woman is advised to undergo an oral glucose tolerance test for further evaluation.

Gestational diabetes (GDM) is a carbohydrate intolerance that is first recognized during pregnancy. GDM occurs in approximately 2% of pregnancies in the UK. Women with GDM are more likely to develop problems with their blood pressure during pregnancy than woman without this condition. In addition, women with GDM may have an increased risk of developing type 2 diabetes later in life.

Babies born to woman with GDM are more likely to be heavy at birth about 4 Kg more. They are at risk of developing low blood glucose levels requiring Special Care Baby Unit admission shortly after birth. There may also be links between GDM in the mother and the development of obesity and type 2 diabetes in the offspring.

GDM during pregnancy used to assist in guiding treatment for women. It may also inform us regarding treating women who have glucose lower than the levels required for diagnosis of GDM. This could prevent the mother developing conditions such as high blood pressure during pregnancy, the baby developing Hypoglycaemia or childhood obesity/type 2 diabetes.

# Giving Birth

The most important factor to choose where to have my baby is safety for me and my baby. To choose the place of birth also choose who will be with and type of care will receive while in labour. It must be the place that feels more comfortable, more relaxed and more in control. Being relaxed is likely to help labour. If anything is upset, you will become tense and may feel more pain.

Occasionally, women develop complications during pregnancy or labour. They need access to specific care that is usually only available in a hospital environment. If a complication arises, it needs to transfer to a consultant unit within a hospital.

The hospital birth care is provided by midwives and obstetricians for high risk. When there are serious experience complications during pregnancy, care is shared with the midwives and the medical team.

My health and well-being will be discussed and evaluated throughout the antenatal period by a midwife, GP and obstetrician. Occasionally care in labour is changed from midwifery-led to obstetric-led care during labour if complications occur.

A home birth may feel more relaxed and in control with a midwife from the team who works in the area where you live with care for you in labour. The midwife met before at antenatal visits or antenatal classes. A water birth can be hired at home birth, but an epidural is not available at home. In case of complication arises, the transfer into the nearest maternity unit by ambulance is needed.

Data from the last decade showed that just under one third of woman who were having their first babies and had planned a home birth transferred into hospital during labour for women having their second or subsequent child, rates range between 1-12%. The most common reasons for transfer were fetal compromise, including meconium stained liquor, and delay in labour. Overall, women having their first baby were two to four times more likely to be transferred during labour than women who had given birth previously.

The rate of postnatal transfer of a maternity unit was about 1.6-3.5% for babies and 1.1-2.8% for women. Even if your baby is born at home, there is a small chance may need to go to hospital. The hospital pediatricians may not be available to offer the post delivery examination, but midwife may be trained to undertake this.

For me, I had an emergency Caesar section after the doctor's team spots my blood pressure is going up. I have no choice of home birth, but it had to be in the hospital only. Also, it had to be in the theater with doctor teams to be ready for the premature baby and my condition. They have to make sure that they have a cot for my baby and have a bed for me.

# Caesarean Section

A Caesarean section is recommended for the satiety of the mother and baby, often advised and performed in certain situations. This procedure performed by an obstetrician trained in the procedure.

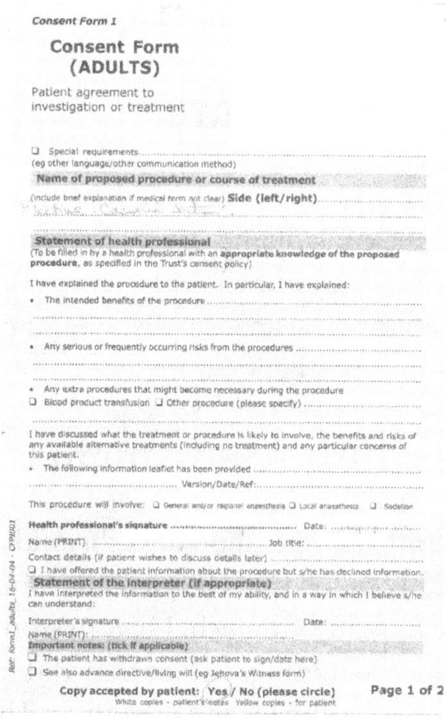

*Consent Form 1*

**Consent Form (ADULTS)**

Patient agreement to investigation or treatment

❑ Special requirements ..........
(eg other language/other communication method)

**Name of proposed procedure or course of treatment**

(include brief explanation if medical term not clear) **Side (left/right)** ..........

**Statement of health professional**

(To be filled in by a health professional with an **appropriate knowledge of the proposed procedure**, as specified in the Trust's consent policy)

I have explained the procedure to the patient. In particular, I have explained:

- The intended benefits of the procedure ..........
- Any serious or frequently occurring risks from the procedures ..........
- Any extra procedures that might become necessary during the procedure

❑ Blood product transfusion ❑ Other procedure (please specify) ..........

I have discussed what the treatment or procedure is likely to involve, the benefits and risks of any available alternative treatments (including no treatment) and any particular concerns of this patient.

- The following information leaflet has been provided ..........

.......... Version/Date/Ref: ..........

This procedure will involve: ❑ General and/or regional anaesthesia ❑ Local anaesthesia ❑ Sedation

**Health professional's signature** .......... Date: ..........

Name (PRINT) .......... Job title: ..........

Contact details (if patient wishes to discuss details later) ..........

❑ I have offered the patient information about the procedure but s/he has declined information.

**Statement of the interpreter (if appropriate)**

I have interpreted the information to the best of my ability, and in a way in which I believe s/he can understand:

Interpreter's signature .......... Date: ..........

Name (PRINT): ..........

**Important notes: (tick if applicable)**

❑ The patient has withdrawn consent (ask patient to sign/date here)

❑ See also advance directive/living will (eg Jehova's Witness form)

**Copy accepted by patient: Yes / No (please circle)** **Page 1 of 2**

White copies - patient's notes Yellow copies - for patient

*Ref: form1_adults_18-04-04 - CFPI001*

Figure 5.1: Consent form

A Caesarean section is when the baby is delivered through an incision (cut) in the abdomen (tummy). A Caesarean may be planned in advance (elective Caesarean section) or be performed at short notice, particularly if there are complications in labour (emergency Caesarean section). An elective Caesarean section is usually performed one week before the baby's due date. This ensures that the baby is sufficiently mature before delivery.

# Before the Procedure

I had been seen at the antenatal clinic by the midwife and the consultants. They checked my medical history; carry out clinical examinations and investigations. The anaesthetist would discuss the choice of the anesthetic for my operation.

# Pre-Operation Assessment

The night before the operation day, the midwife came to take my blood sample, gave me tablets to reduce the acid in my stomach. I had to stop eating or drinking before midnight since they did not know for sure what time is my operation. This is to ensure that my stomach is empty and if I was to vomit while under anaesthesia, I will not inhale food particles that could damage my lungs. My case will be inserted in the theatre between the schedule operations. Therefore, nobody knows when the theatre room will be available.

In the morning the midwife gave me a hospital gown, a pair of special socks for preventing blood clot and she checks my wrist band with my personal details again. The midwife, my husband and I walked to the theatre together. My husband changed clothes when we arrived there.

# During the Procedure

My husband can be present during the Caesarean section since I had an epidural or spinal anaesthesia and I was awake. However, if I had a general anesthetic, my husband would have to leave the theatre.

Most caesarean sections are done under regional anaesthesia with sensation of the lower body is numb. This is usually safer for mother and baby. There are three types of regional anaesthesia:

**Spinal:** It is the most commonly used in both planned and emergency operations. Local anesthetic and pain relieving drugs is injected inside a bag of fluid inside the backbone which the nerves and spinal cord that carry feeling from the lower body and control muscle movement.

**Epidural:** A thin plastic tube is placed outside the bag of fluid near the nerves carrying pain from the uterus. It can be topped up with stronger local anesthetic. In an epidural a larger dose of local anesthetic is needed than in a spinal and it takes longer to work.

**Combined spinal-epidural:** The spinal can be used for the caesarean section. The epidural can be used to give more anesthetic and pain relieving drugs after the operation.

Advantages of regional anaesthesia compared with general anaesthesia are the spinals and epidurals are safer for mother and baby, the mother will not be sleepy afterwards and have good pain relief afterwards and the baby will be born more alert. However, the spinals and epidurals can lower the blood pressure. This is easily treated with the fluids given through the drip and by giving drugs to raise the blood pressure. It may cause itching, shaky, headache and tingling down one leg.

I had a regional anesthetic done in the operating theatre while my husband sits next to me. Acanula, the dip, was placed in a vein in my wrist with some local anesthetic. The equipment to monitor my blood pressure and heart rate were attached.

I was asked to lie on my side, curling my back. The anesthetist cleans my back with sterilising solution. Then, she would find a suitable point between two of the nines in the middle of my back and inject local anesthetic to numb the skin.

Then, for a spinal, a fine needle is passed through this numb area and into the spinal fluid. I felt a tingling going down one leg. Then a local anesthetic and a pain relieving drug were injected. For an epidural, a larger needle is needed to allow the epidural catheter to be threaded into the epidural space. I know the spinal or epidural is working when my leg begin to feel tingly, heavy and numb. The numbness spread gradually up my body. The anaesthetist is checked with a cold spray if it is ready for the operation.

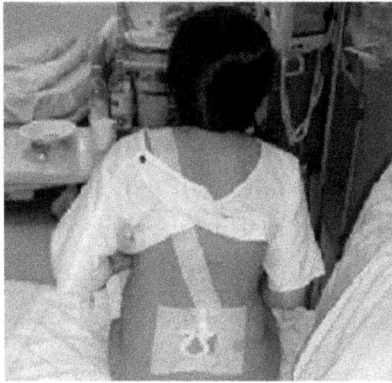

Figure 5.2: Anaesthesia location

Then, they have a screen separated us from the surgeons While my husband sits next to my head on the left and the anaesthetist stay on my right side and keep checking the machine reading my blood pressure, heart and other monitoring machine. A midwife inserts a urinary catheter into my bladder to keep it empty during the operation.

While I was anaesthetized, the obstetrician made a small incision in my skin above pubic bone. She then made a second incision into the lower section of my uterus. I feel pulling and pressure in my stomach but I do not feel pain.

The obstetrician said she can see my transplant kidney on the left side of my tummy. Then, I heard a baby's crying. My baby was delivered and passes to midwife. Pediatricians examine him in the cot on the far side of the theatre. She brings him over to let me see him and lets my husband take a picture. After the checking, he went straight to the special care baby unit because the baby was small and very premature.

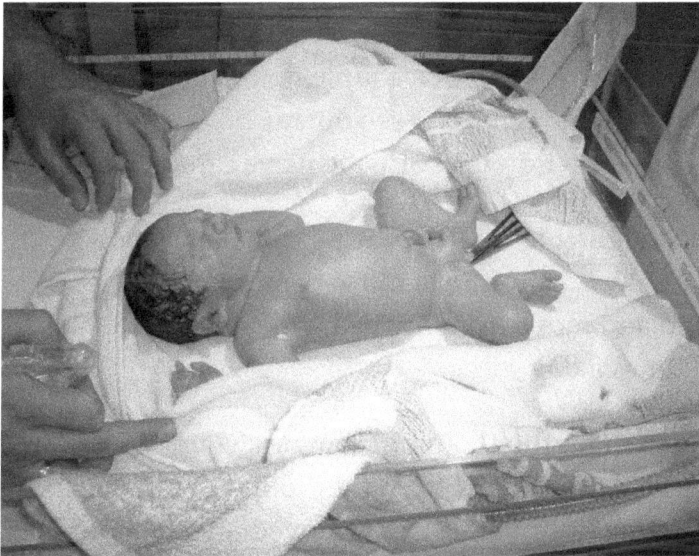

Figure 5.3: First picture 12 minutes old

They give me a drug Syntocinon which put into my drip to help my uterus contract and deliver the placenta. An antibiotic is also routinely given to reduce the chance of wound infection. While the placenta is delivered, the obstetrician closed the incision. Each layer of muscle and skin that has been cut, then needs to be closed using sutures (stitches), staples or clips. At the end of the operation, they give me a pain relieving suppository.

# After the Procedure

I was transferred to the recovery room to monitor my blood pressure for a couple hours to ensure everything is well. I can see my husband around, but my baby is in the baby intensive care.

I feel tingling in my leg when a spinal anesthetic gradually wear off. The nurse comes to help me stand and move from my bed. I have pain relieving 3-4 times a day.

I had a drain tube coming from my wound. This collected tissue fluid from the wound in a small collecting chamber. It was removed after 24 hours. The catheter was left in position for 12 -24 hours until I was more mobile.

I had a small sip of water after the procedure and have food when I feel well enough. I had to up on my feet within 24 hours of a Caesarean section. The midwife gave me some pain killers and helped me moved around. A physiotherapist came to see me and discussed about the post-natal exercises.

The main risks of Caesarean section are development of heavy bleeding at the time of surgery, injury to other organs, infection in the wound or bladder after delivery; this can be controlled with antibiotics, development of a thrombosis (blood clot) in the leg veins after delivery and risks for subsequent pregnancies include: placenta prevails where the placenta lies in the lower part of the uterus.

Born from Kidney Transplant Mother

# Chapter 6

# Neonatal Equipment

## Transferring Mothers and Babies

The pregnancy may be complicated by any form of emergency. Few people consider the possibility that their baby could be born some weeks before the due date. They may need to be given special care for the first few days, weeks or months after the birth.

Some circumstances may need to transfer to another hospital.

## Special Care

Sometimes babies are born early or doctor may decide that baby needs to be delivered early. In these cases the baby may need to be cared for in our neonatal intensive care unit or NICU.

It is difficult decisions to make because we are sensitive to the impact that transfer to another hospital.

Decision sometimes have to be made at short notice, but are always made by a consultant obstetrician and consultant pediatricians and a management plan put in place.

Studies have shown that it is much safer and that babies have better outcomes if babies are born where there are appropriate and already available facilities rather than wait for delivery and transfer to an available cot as a new born baby.

The obstetrician will have direct communication with the nearest appropriate receiving hospital and transport will be arranged. Transport has been almost always by ambulance with a midwife to accompany to the receiving hospital.

When arriving at the receiving hospital, the cares will be fully taken over by a new obstetric team and the plan of care may change at that point. The urine and blood samples may be needed.

When the threat of the premature baby in labour or delivery process has gone, then the antenatal care will be continuing as before.

# Neonatal intensive care unit (NICU)

Instruments and Equipment for premature baby in the neonatal unit gives babies the best chance of survival and a healthy future.

## Incubators

Premature baby's place inside an incubator will help to keep them warm which are the basic need for the baby.

The temperature inside the incubator can be controlled by manually or automatically respond from the baby's temperature. There is a small sensor on the baby skin to tell the baby's temperature. If the sensor drops off and does not read the baby's temperature. It will sound the alarm to the baby's nurse.

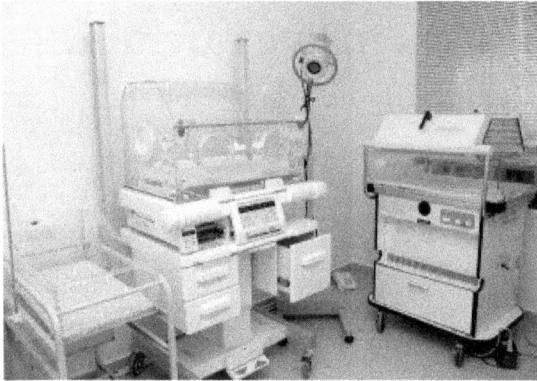

Figure 6.1: Incubators to warm the baby

# Vital sign monitors

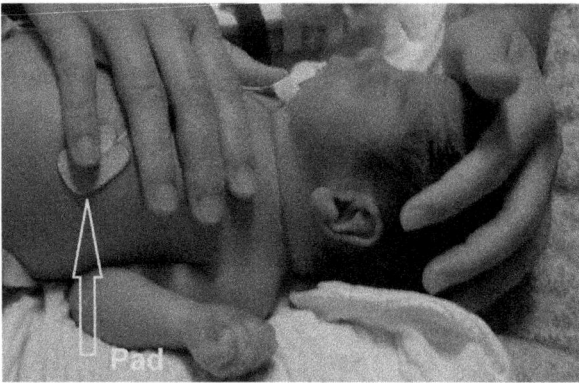

Figure 6.2: Pad on the baby chest monitors the breathing

The small pads may be placed on the baby's chest. The pads can detect changes during breathing and pauses in breathing. The pads pick up the electrical signals given out by the baby's heart. It also checks it is beating properly. This may trigger the alarm.

# Blood Gas Monitors

The blood gas monitor is a sensor which shines light through the skin of the baby. It is normally strapped gently to the baby's foot or hand. This sensor monitors the amount of oxygen in the baby's blood.

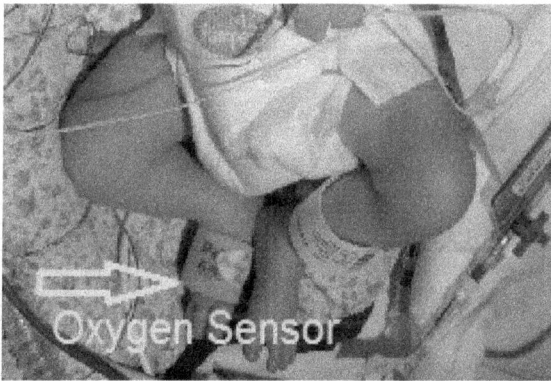

Figure 6.3: sensor monitors the amount of oxygen

# Intravenous Line

This is a thin plastic tube place inside one of the baby's veins. This allows doctors to give drugs such as antibiotics directly into the blood stream.

The doctors may choose a vein in the baby's arm, leg or the umbilical cord.

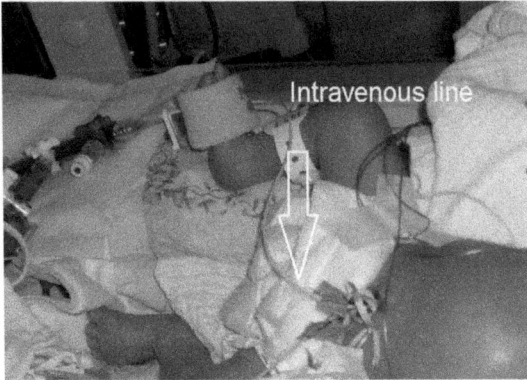

Figure 6.4: Intravenous line in the baby's line

# Long Lines

This is a very fine tube. This may be fed into a vein to let staff give nutrition in case the baby is too premature or unwell to take food or fluids through the baby's mouth. This line can also be used for injecting medication.

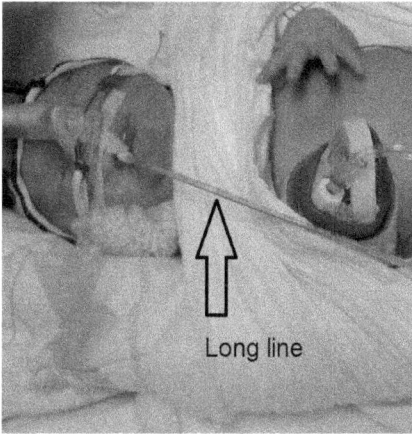

Figure 6.5: Long line position

# Larger Tube

The doctor may place a large tube into an artery to allow them to take blood samples. They may choose artery in the arm, leg or umbilical cord.

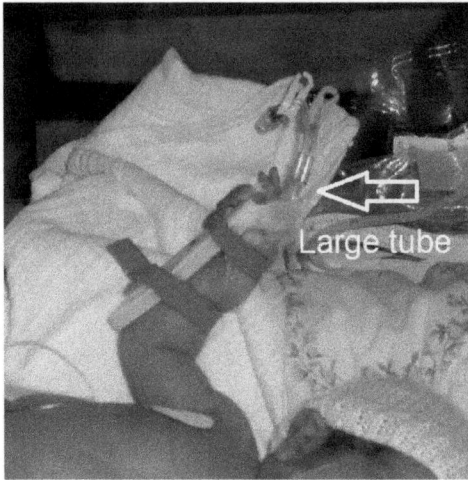

Figure 6.6: Large tube

# Gentle Breathing Support

A continuous Positive Airway Pressure (CPAP) helps the baby's breath with air flow with slightly raises the pressure and helps the baby's lungs inflated. Some babies need a little helps with their breathing, but do not need a ventilator.

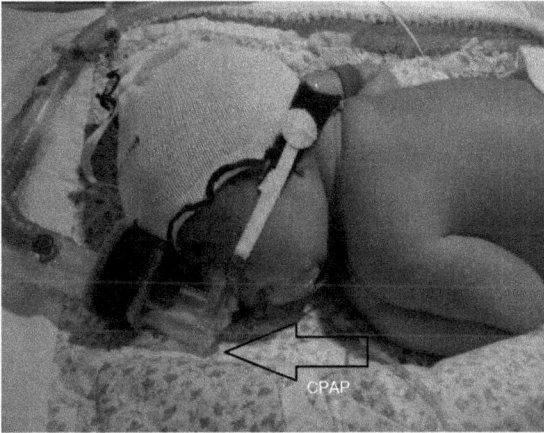

Figure 6.7: Continuous Positive Airway Pressure (CPAP)

# Ventilators and Surfactant

This machine drives air through a tube placed into the baby's windpipe, which is called the trachea. There are two types:

- Positive pressure ventilators blow oxygen gently into the baby's lung through a tube that is passed through the baby's mouth or nose. The rate will be regularly adjusted to meet the baby's need. This sophisticated machine is designed to inflate the lungs and reduce damage to the baby's lungs.

- High frequency ventilators puff small amounts of air into the lungs hundreds of times a minute. This is a natural process that is like the panting style of breathing.

When the baby is in the mother's womb, a baby receives all of the oxygen from the mother's blood. It passes to the baby's blood in the placenta before travelling to the baby through the umbilical cord.

When the baby was born, they have to breathe to get oxygen into their body. This can be a problem for very premature babies because their lungs may not be fully developed; the babies may be well and very weak.

If the baby's lungs are not fully developed, the doctors may use a tube to pass surfactant directly into the baby's lungs. The surfactant helps to reduce the tension on the surface of the lungs. This makes breathing easier for the baby.

When the baby is taken off a ventilator, the baby may breathe well for a bit and then become tired. The doctor will replace the ventilator and try again later, the periods off the ventilator should increase.

When the baby's blood oxygen level drops and the baby's chest does not move in time with the ventilator, the breathing tube may be blocked with mucus. The staff may give the baby a chance to breathe before replace the tube.

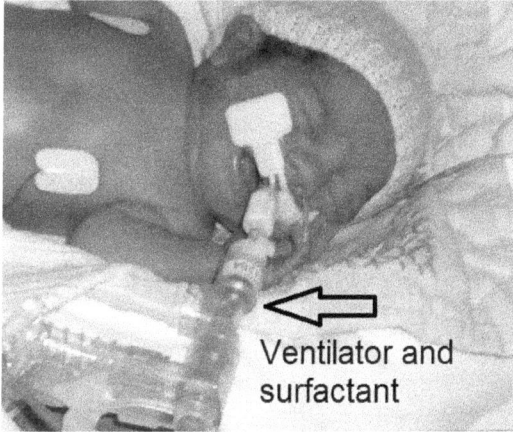

Figure 6.8: Ventilator and surfactant

# Apnea Alarms

When the ventilator has been removed, the baby may take a pause in their breathing. However, babies may be fitted with monitor to check if they are breathing regularly. If the baby pauses for too long between two breaths, the alarm will set off.

Born from Kidney Transplant Mother

# Chapter 7

# Premature Medical Procedure

Most babies in the neonatal unit need tests and procedures. These causes short-term mild discomfort, but not long-term risk. The medical staff has a responsibility to discuss with the mother. She understands the reason for any tests and treatment being given to the baby. However, in case of low risk procedures, the parents will not be formally asked for consent. The low risk is the procedure might not harm the baby.

## Pain Relief

The neonatal units have a policy to provide pain relief for the baby as much as possible because the babies feel pain. The parents can comfort the baby by practicing containment holding.

The following procedures the parents will not be asked for consent for staff to carry out.

# Blood Test

Blood acts as the body's transport system carries oxygen around the body, moving nutrients, waste products and chemical. It is packed with living cells and these cells give clues about the baby's overall health. Analysing a sample of blood can give many of information about what is going on inside a baby. Samples are taken by pricking the skin from the back of the hand or the heel. These pricks leave tiny scars, but do not affect the growth of the hand or foot.

## Blood Test - Sugar Levels

Doctors want to know that the baby is managing to control the amount of sugar in the baby's blood. Blood needs to contain enough sugar to distribute energy to all the body's organs. The baby may need supplements through the intravenous tubes. Babies with low birth weight or born to diabetic mothers, may have problems maintaining blood sugar levels and need monitoring.

# Blood Test - Gases

The blood transportation system carries oxygen from the lungs to organs and carries carbon dioxide from the organs to the lungs.

Measuring the amount of these gases along with levels of acid can give clues about how well the baby is breathing. It also indicates if kidneys work as the baby's needs.

# Blood Test - Platelets

The platelets play a part in preventing excessive bleeding. In premature a number often reduced, doctors may transfuse if the levels are very low.

# Blood Test - Haemoglobin

Haemoglobin is the chemical that blood uses transport oxygen. The babies become anaemic if they have too few red blood cells. The oxygen carried to the organs may be low. Therefore, the doctors may give a blood transfusion.

# Blood Test - White Blood Cells

The role of the white blood cells is fighting infections. If the level of the white blood cells in the baby's blood is very low, doctors can give drugs to the baby to help to produce more.

# Lumbar Puncture

In case the baby has a severe infection, doctors may want to take samples of fluid that surrounds the spinal cord. A doctor will use a needle to insert between bones, low in the baby's back. This fluid flows down from the brain. This liquid can show if the infection is in this vital part of the nervous system.

# Phototherapy for Jaundice

Blood cells live in the body for a few days or weeks, then they are broken down and new ones are formed. A chemical called "bilirubin" is released when the blood cells break down. The premature babies and newborn babies with liver problems cannot remove it fast enough. If the level of bilirubin is very high in the blood, it could cause brain damage. Premature babies are placed under a blue light because bilirubin is broken by blue light. In case of the bilirubin levels is too high, the doctors may exchange transfusion to replace the baby's blood with fresh bilirubin-free blood.

# Eye Tests

If a baby is born too early, then their retinal blood vessels do not develop completely which can cause problems. Abnormal blood vessels may grow out of the retina and cause scar tissue to form, leading to detachment of the retina. The retina is found at the back of the eye and is a very complex and sensitive structure that is responsible for the initial formation of the visual image. The light image is transferred by the optic nerve to the brain, which allows us to see.

Premature babies are at risk of having problems with their eyes. In case of the babies was born with weighed less than 1500 g or less than 32 weeks, the ophthalmologist regularly examines the retina at the back of the baby's eyes. If the premature babies have a condition called Retinopathy of Prematurity (ROP) with affect the retinas. Then, tests and special treatment are carried out on the unit.

# Hearing Test

Premature babies may have a greater risk of hearing problems than full term babies. Therefore, all babies will have a hearing test before leaving hospital.

# Head Ultrasound Scan

Doctors use the head ultrasound scan to see the structure of baby's brain, check if there are bleeding or other problems.

# Endotracheal Tubes

The endotracheal tube is the tube placed in the windpipe for ventilation. Sometimes these tubes fall out or blocked, the staff can replace without consent the baby's parents.

# Medical Procedures Requiring Consent

There are procedures may have a risk for the baby or long-term effect. The staff will discuss with parents in advance. You may need to give signature as evidence of the agreement. It is important that parents understand what is being done and the implications of what may happen. In an emergency they may not have time to discuss the procedure beforehand, but they will talk through afterwards.

Staff needs a parent's permission for the following procedures:

# MRI Scan

The MRI generates pictures of organs inside a baby without harming the baby. The baby may need to be in a stable condition and placed in a special incubator before MRI procedure.

# Special Blood Tests

The special blood test needs to screen a baby for viral infections, genetic testing and surgical procedure.

# Intravenous Lines

These lines usually provide fluid or giving important medication like antibiotics. This occasionally can break the delicate blood vessels or blocked. The fluids can leak into the surrounding tissues, causing swelling or damage the skin leaving a scar.

## Long Lines

This is a special fine line passed into one of the large veins of the baby to give nutrition. However, it is not easy to sit in the right place. Therefore, it may be blocked or leak if it is not correct, but the staff will watch carefully and remove them if there are any concerns.

## Umbilical Catheters

The fine tubes inserted into blood vessels in the tummy button. In the artery is used for measuring blood pressure and sampling blood gases. The vein is used for giving nutrition and medicines. If they leak, the baby may lose some blood and a transfusion may be needed.

## Pneumothorax and Chest Drains

When the premature babies are being ventilated, some air may leak from damaged air sacs in the lungs. Air bubbles may form in the lung tissues or around the lungs forming a pneumothorax. Large pockets of air can compress the lungs and make it work more difficult. The baby is given a local anaesthetic when doctor passes a small tube through the chest wall letting the air escape.

# Immunisations

A routine immunisations will start at 8 weeks after birth. This needs parents' consent/agreement. Immunisation for baby's first 18 months.

DIP/TERT/PERT/HIB/Polio : at 2 months old

MEN C : at 2 months old

DIP/TERT/PERT/HIB/Polio : at 3 months old

MEN C : at 3 months old

DIP/TERT/PERT/HIB/Polio : at 4 months old

MEN C : at 4 months old

MMR : at 13 months old

MMR : at 3-5 years old

# Infection

Sometimes infections are caused by germs collecting on long lines or ventilation tubing in the windpipe. Premature babies have little ability to fight infection and it needs treatment.

# Significant Medical Problems

The baby may have some weaknesses or problems which cause the baby were born early.

# Brain Haemorrhage

The small haemorrhages may not cause long term problems. When the tiny vessels in some areas of a developing baby's brain leak and bleeding, this can turn to blood clots and block the flow from the brain to the spinal cord. When the large bleeds occur, it may limit blood and oxygen flow to certain areas of the brain. This will cause the cells die. Doctors will monitor and carry out regular ultrasound scans when there is large bleeds.

# Patent Ductus

The connection between the vessels supplying blood to the lungs and the vessels supplying blood to the body normally closes within hours of birth for a full term baby. This can still open with premature babies who born early or can be reopened if the baby gets an infection. This condition can detect from ultrasound scan. Doctors may give drugs to help close it or may need an operation.

# Heart defects

It is urgent to transfer the baby with heart problem to a cardiac center. They may have to be in a neonatal unit until they grew big enough for surgery.

Born from Kidney Transplant Mother

# Chapter 8

# Neonatal Care

Technology and advances in medical care means that we can now look after babies born very early in pregnancy babies sick at birth. The neonatal unit in the hospital wards specially designed and equipped to care for sick newborn babies.

Few people consider the possibility that their baby could be born many weeks before the due date. They may need to be given special care. Some babies are admitted to the neonatal unit because they have an infection, need intravenous antibiotics, need extra monitoring, need breathing support and they may have serious jaundice.

Occasionally doctors may have found an abnormality; the baby will need an operation. In that case the baby may need to be transferred to a specialist hospital.

Most babies are in the neonatal unit since they were born weeks before their due date. The length of a baby's stay varies from days to months and depends on each baby's needs.

The neonatal units are staffed for 24 hours a day. All people entering the neonatal units will be obliged to wash their hands and forearms with a special disinfectant. Then, apply an anti-bacterial gel in order to reduce the chances of babies being infected by bacteria or infection from outside of the unit.

Many babies in the neonatal unit are extremely tiny and immature. The room is full of monitors, high-tech equipment and the frequent sound of alarm. The displays are often designed to be easily seen and grab attention. The equipment that surrounds them is designed to keep them warm, to monitor many of their body's functions and to support their breathing. All of the equipment can be distracting.

# Baby Arrive Early

There are many reasons that babies born premature:

- Pregnancies with twins, triplets or more: The babies may be small and they may need a lot of support.

- Infection and involving the sac around the baby in the womb triggered the delivery.

- Stressful can cause labour early such as the death of a relative or friend, moving home and long distance travel.

- Mother's waters break early and starting the delivery process. If labour starts while a baby are less than 35 weeks, the doctor will give two sets of drugs. The first one is to delay the labour for a day or two. The second one is to help the baby's lungs to mature quickly so that they will function better after delivery.

- Emergency: it may be the mother started to bleed or had high blood pressure, some problem with the umbilical cord and problem with the placenta.

- Pre-Eclampsia: it affects 1 in 14 pregnancies and cause one in three of premature births. It can be dangerous because it develops rapidly. The main symptoms are headaches, swollen feet and high blood pressure. The only way to stop pre-eclampsia is to deliver the baby early.

- Baby is not growing well in the womb: this can find out from the antenatal screening test. This causes from there was not enough blood flowing to and from the placenta. If the doctor believes that the baby is going to be safer outside the womb, they would advise to have the baby delivered early and it may be recommended a caesarean section. This is because it is less stress on the baby.

# Care Levels

There are 3 levels of care units in the special care which depends on the condition of the babies such as very young, very small and sick.

- Intensive care (NICU) – Level 3: The whole range of medical neonatal care.

- High dependency – Level 2: This case involves some breathing support and intravenous nutrition.

- Special care baby units (SCBU) – Level 1: This involves some tube-feeding, additional oxygen support and light therapy (phototherapy).

# Transferring from Unit to Unit

The specialist transport teams will give support during the transfer with a high-tech transport incubator which is capable of full intensive care support through the journey.

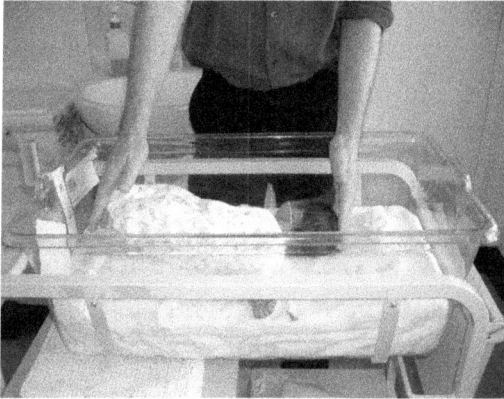

Figure 8.1: Infant incubator

# Transitional Care

This involves some process of intravenous antibiotics in a postnatal ward and preparing a baby to go home.

# Quiet Times

Neonatal units have quiet times to give the baby time to rest. The lights will be dimmed and curtains drawn. During this time there will be less disturbed babies as little as possible.

# Doctor's Round

The morning round, the staff will plan for the baby's care. The evening round allows the daytime and nigh time staffs to coordinate their care.

# Cares

There are different types of nurses, including neonatal nurses, advanced neonatal practitioners (ANNP's) and nurse consultants.

- Ward manager: look after baby's welfare and safety. Her team composites of nursing sisters, staff nurses, midwives, nursery nurses, ward clerk and housekeeper.

- Neonatologist and pediatrics consultant will see and give baby treatment when it is needed. The lead consultant of the pediatrics doctors is specialist registrars and senior house officers.

- Pre-registration house officers and medical students may present in a teaching hospital.

- Physiotherapists will help baby's physical development.

- Dietitians will make sure that baby gets the best diet.

- Pharmacists will look after medicines that are prescribed to babies.

- The ophthalmologist will check babies' eyes.

- Audiology technicians will check babies' hearing.

- Radiological technicians will do the X-rays.

- Neonatal consultant or radiological will do an ultrasound.

- Electronic medical engineers and technicians will maintain the high technology equipment.

# Take Part in Baby Care

The staff may do most of the work and over the next few days the staff will encourage parents to become involved and understand what is what happen in their baby.

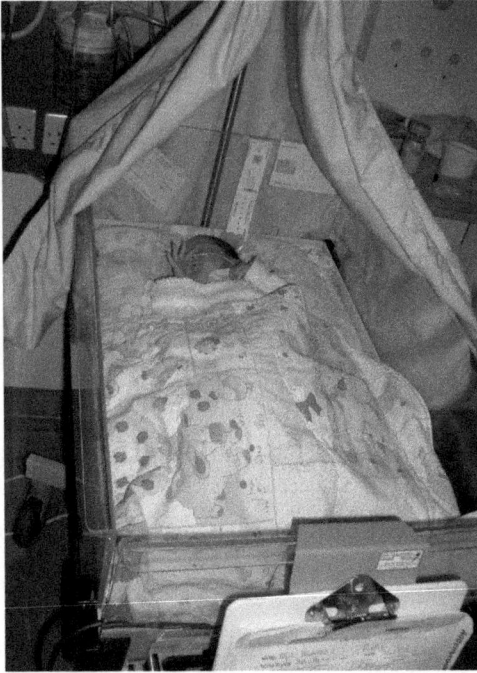

Figure 8.2: Bed in special neonatal unit

The premature baby can tell many things and we can communicate messages of love and reassurance to the baby by observing the body language and reactions, to get to know, to understand and support the baby's growth and development.

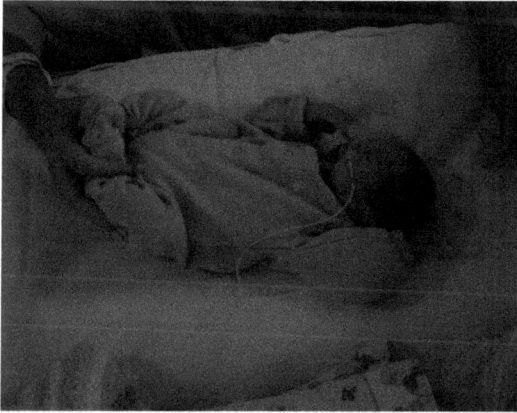

Figure 8.3: In comfortable position

The premature baby feels comfortable when he has her hands near face or mouth, the body is curled up position and so are the arms and legs, have feet together, smiling and relaxed expression.

The premature baby feel uncomfortable when he is thrust arms and legs rigidly into the air, arching his back, frowning or scowling, spreading the fingers and toes out, moaning or crying, yawning or hiccoughs during treatment and look away.

# Alarming Noises

Each piece of equipment is fitted with alarms that are designed to warn the staff of any problems. These alarms are very sensitive and are often triggered by the baby. There is different between normal, routine alarm noises and the ones that mean the baby needs more immediate help. The staff will respond to these quickly.

# Baby Appearance

Many premature babies have a fine covering of dark hair when they are born; it is called "lanugo". It stimulated by the baby receiving some of the mother's hormones, while in the womb. The skin could seem waxy and it can be transparent. This is because there is little or no fat beneath it. A fine network of blood vessels can be seen through the baby's skin. The baby may only be the length of your hand and sleep almost 20 hours per day.

The skull bones of premature babies are quite soft. A soft pillow or a water pillow may prevent a flattened head shape if the head lies on the hard flat surface for long. When the baby is mature enough to go home the skull bones will have hardened up and a pillow is not needed.

By the time that the baby reaches the expected date to be born, the baby is unlikely to look very different from a full term baby of the same weight.

# See Baby for the First Time

If the doctor delivered babies by caesarean section, it could take a few days before the mother can see the baby. Friends and family can visit the baby and bring some photos to show the mother.

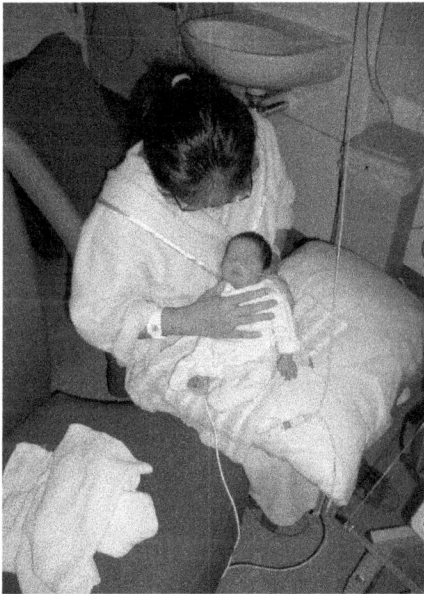

Figure 8.4: Mother holds the premature baby

It is important that baby gets to know the mother, hears the mother's voice and mother's scent. It is good for parents to spend time talking to and touching baby while the staffs try to handle the baby as little as possible. The staff constantly checks the monitors. Therefore, mother can spend time watching the baby.

## Containment Holding

This containment holding can help the baby feel secure, relaxed and loved. The baby may be much more comfortable left lying in the incubator and the staff may suggest that mother's touch the baby if they think the baby is well enough. Place one hand firmly but gently on the baby's head and the other hand on the baby's middle. At this stage the baby will enjoy a still hold more than stroking or patting which can be over-stimulating. To reduce the chance of introducing an infection into the incubator, always roll up sleeves, remove wrist watches or jewelry before wash and dry your hands and lower arms.

## Caring Touch

Some medical procedures can cause your baby discomfort. To help the baby feel more comfortable and secure, the parents are the best to give the baby this support by reassuring touch. There are various ways to comfort the baby. The doctors and nurses will show which is the most appropriate. This is depended on how stressed of the baby. If the baby is so tired, the staff will suggest keeping contact to a minimum.

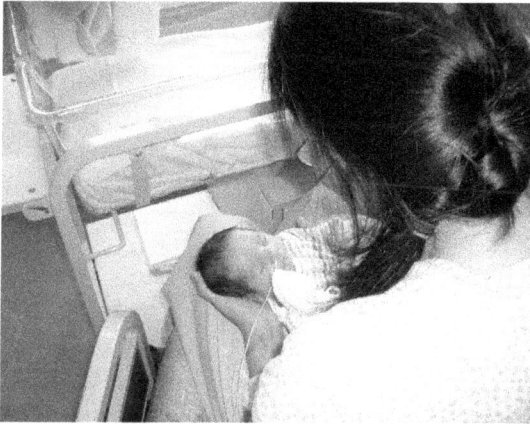

Figure 8.5: Caring touch from the mother

# Kangaroo Care

Kangaroo care is the first times parents feel that they are really having contact with the baby. It is a great way of establishing a lasting attachment. The baby receives very much comfort that this contact can have a very positive effect on the baby's health.

If the baby is well enough, the mother may be able to lift the baby out of the incubator to snuggle gently on her chest. It is the best if the baby can lie directly on her skin. This gives a wonderful feeling of contact between mother and baby. This also helps to keep the baby warm and calm a baby's breathing. It has to be careful not pull any of the cables or tubes that may be attached to the baby.

Kangaroo care can improve the amount of oxygen in the baby's blood. The baby tends to cry less and sleep more deeply, which supports the baby's health and development.

# Nappy Changing

This is a good way to do routine tasks and take an active parents' role in baby's day to day care.

# Feeding

Feeding the baby is a superb way of helping care as it is the time when the baby is likely to be awake.

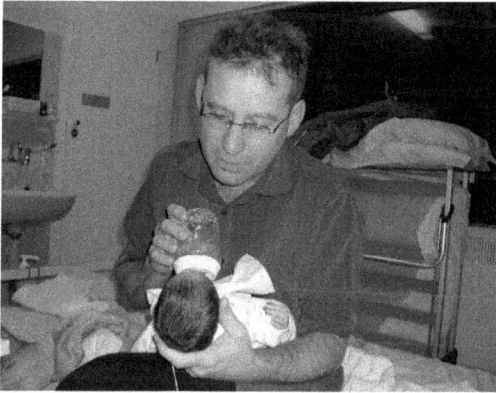

Figure 8.6: Feeding

# Bathing

The washing, even with warm water, could cool the baby down. Therefore, the nurses may be reluctant to wash the baby. The waxy 'Vemix' from life in the womb will do no harm and are best left where they are. Once the baby has grown a little and is stronger, mother may be able to join in with the fun of bath.

# New Daddy

Father can join in with caring for the baby in the same way as mothers, including feeding, bathing, nappy changing, kangaroo care and containment holding. This can help daddy and baby get to know each other. It also takes some of the pressure off from the mother.

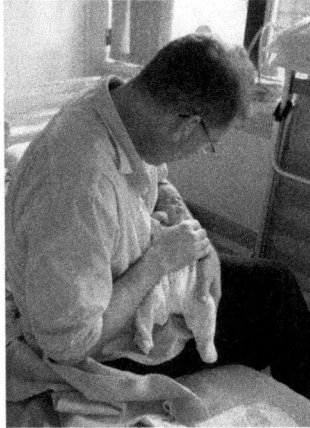

Figure 8.7: Father holds the premature baby

# Chapter 9

# Premature Feeding

When the baby is in the mother's womb, the baby got nutrients and fluid via the placenta and umbilical cord. The are many ways to feed the premature baby. This depends on the baby's health and maturity.

## Artificial feeding Total Parenteral Nutrition (TPN)

This TPN is for babies whose stomach and gut are not developed enough to digest food or the baby is not very well.

The mixture contains glucose, salts and water, with amino acids, fats, vitamins and minerals can be dripped directly into a baby's blood stream from the long fine tube into a vein in the arm or leg.

# Tube –Feeding

Premature babies cannot coordinate the muscles needed for swallowing. They can take food into their stomach by the naso-gastric tube through their noses and down into their stomach.

When the milk feed via the tube, the babies can practice their sucking at the same time as receiving a tube feed.

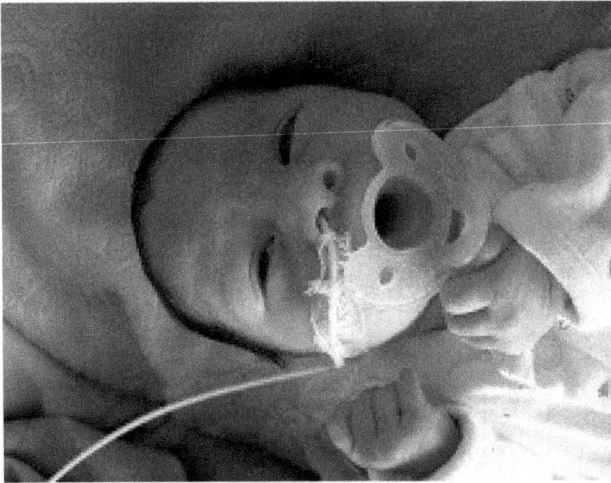

Figure 9.1: Premature dummy to learn sucking

# Supplemented Feeds

The first milk mothers produce is called colostrum, which contains a lot of infection-fighting proteins and cells. The kidney transplant mother cannot breast feeding because all chemicals pass from a mother's blood to breast milk. Her milk will contain traces of anti-rejection elements medication. Therefore, the supplement colostrum in the formula milk is necessary. The baby will receive enough energy and fluid to get well quickly.

# Fortification

Premature babies may need dietary needs differ. Some may need extra protein, minerals and vitamins. Therefore, they may need to add fortifiers in the formula milk.

# Neonatal Vitamins

- Dalavit: 0.3 mls daily via oral syringe from day 2 - 12 months of age.

- Sytron: 1 ml daily via oral syringe from 4 weeks - 12 months of age.

Coombs positive babies (jaundiced) receive Folic acid 1 ml (0.5 mgs) until weaned.

# Bottle Feeding

Babies are given formula specially designed for premature babies. A specially designed bottle that hold 25-50 ml with a special teat will be provided for a baby who can coordinate breathing, sucking and swallowing. The dietitian will recommend specific dietary needs for individual babies.

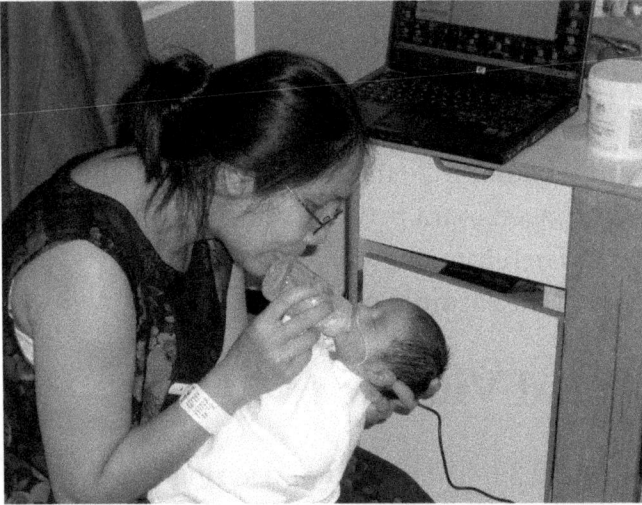

Figure 9.2 : Milk bottle for premature babies

# Going Home

When the baby is stable enough not to need the specialist help in the neonatal unit and the staff on the unit believes that the babies are well enough to leave the hospital and their parents are capable of looking after them and their parents can provide all aspects of the baby's care. Then, it is time to go home.

The baby should be able to maintain a body temperature just like the full term baby. The best temperature is around 18 degree C.

# Travelling Home

Transporting the baby home, even on the shortest of journeys always uses a suitable car seat.

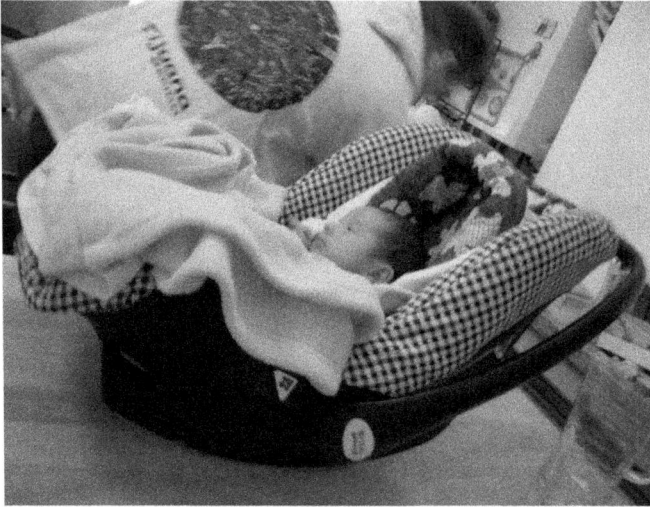

Figure 9.3: Car seat for premature babies

# Respiratory Syncytial Virus (RSV)

RSV can cause cold-like symptoms, breathing difficulties if the lungs are affected. For premature baby is getting lung infections, the baby could be at great risk of being seriously ill if infected with RSV.

# Long term Medical Problems

Premature babies spent a long time on a ventilator can become wheezy when they get a cold or virus that affects their chests. Others may have later learning or movement difficulties.

# Checking Baby's Health

When any problems develop, the doctor should have seen the baby or should take the baby to the nearest hospital emergency department. Signs that baby becoming unwell are as follows:

- Feverish, fretful

- Reluctant and disinterested to feed

- Vomiting

- Change in stools, more frequent, loose, watery and explosive.

- Not as responsive as usual, awakens less readily.

- Seem more floppy than usual.

- Breathing more rapid, noisy, or there may be long pauses between some breaths.

- More pale than usual.

- Blotchy skin, rash that does not become much lighter when a glass tumbler is pressed against it. This is possibly serious and need urgently help.

# Travel Abroad

Most of travel vaccines can be given over four weeks. It also needs to be immunized against other diseases such as yellow fever. In case of travelling to tropical countries, it needs protection against malaria. There is no immunization against malaria, but the doctor is able to give advice on taking anti-malarial drugs.

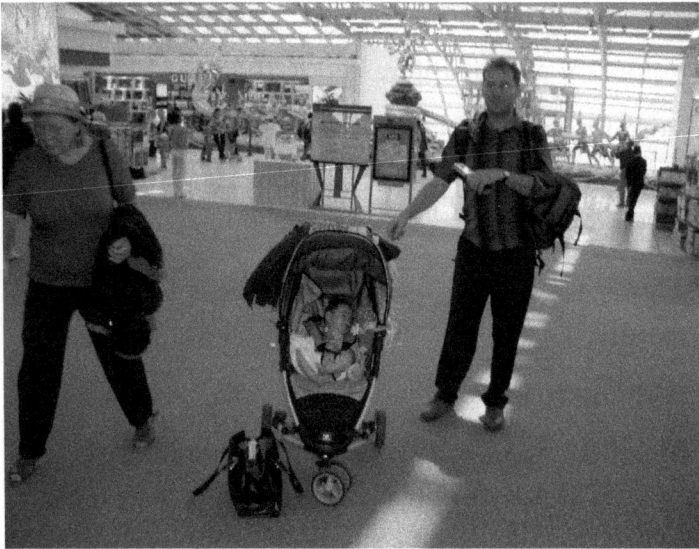

Figure 9.4: In the airport

# Chapter 10

# Immunisation for

# Premature

We take our baby home and then we take him to see the GP and health visitor for immunisation. Despite the baby was born premature but the immunisation programmed begins at 2, 3, 4 months. The immunisations DTP (diphtheria, tetanus and pertussis or whooping cough) and Hib (Haemophilus influenza type B) which are given as one injection and polio is given as drops by mouth. The premature baby may receive the immunisations while still in the NICU or SCBU unit.

## Immunisation at Home

At Neonatal intensive care unit, parents need to consent for immunizations of neonates (BCG). The health professional has discussed with us about the procedure, the intended benefits of the procedure, how the vaccination will be given, potential risk factors and contraindications, any likely side effects of the vaccination and any alternative procedure that are available,

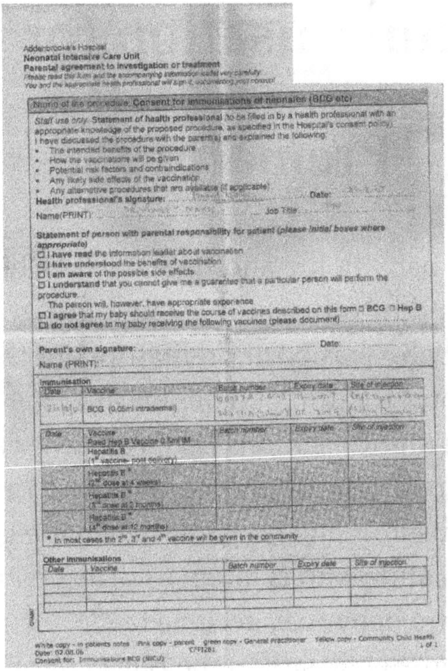

Addenbrooke's Hospital
**Neonatal Intensive Care Unit**
**Parental agreement to investigation or treatment**
*Please read this form and the accompanying information leaflet very carefully.*
*You and the appropriate health professional will sign it, documenting your consent.*

Name of the procedure: **Consent for immunisations of neonates (BCG etc)**

*Staff use only*: **Statement of health professional** (to be filled in by a health professional with an appropriate knowledge of the proposed procedure, as specified in the Hospital's consent policy)
I have discussed the procedure with the parent(s) and explained the following:

- The intended benefits of the procedure
- How the vaccinations will be given
- Potential risk factors and contraindications
- Any likely side effects of the vaccination
- Any alternative procedures that are available (if applicable)

**Health professional's signature:** ............ Date: ............
Name(PRINT): ............ Job Title ............

**Statement of person with parental responsibility for patient** (*please initial boxes where appropriate*)
☐ **I have read** the information leaflet about vaccination
☐ **I have understood** the benefits of vaccination
☐ **I am aware** of the possible side effects
☐ **I understand** that you cannot give me a guarantee that a particular person will perform the procedure.
The person will, however, have appropriate experience
☐ **I agree** that my baby should receive the course of vaccines described on this form ☐ **BCG** ☐ **Hep B**
☐ **I do not agree** to my baby receiving the following vaccines (please document) ............

**Parent's own signature:** ............ Date: ............
Name (PRINT): ............

**Immunisation**

| Date | Vaccine | Batch number | Expiry date | Site of injection |
|---|---|---|---|---|
| | BCG (0.05ml intradermal) | | | |

| Date | Vaccine<br>Paed Hep B Vaccine 0.5ml IM | Batch number | Expiry date | Site of injection |
|---|---|---|---|---|
| | Hepatitis B (1st vaccine- post delivery) | | | |
| | Hepatitis B * (2nd dose at 4 weeks) | | | |
| | Hepatitis B * (3rd dose at 2 months) | | | |
| | Hepatitis B * (4th dose at 12 months) | | | |

* In most cases the 2nd, 3rd and 4th vaccine will be given in the community

**Other immunisations**

| Date | Vaccine | Batch number | Expiry date | Site of injection |
|---|---|---|---|---|
| | | | | |
| | | | | |
| | | | | |
| | | | | |

White copy - in patients notes Pink copy - parent green copy - General Practitioner Yellow copy - Community Child Health
Date: 02.08.06 CF1281 1 of 1
Consent for: Immunisations BCG (NICU)

Figure 10.1: Consent form for immunization of neonates

The reactions to the immunisations, which the premature baby may develop are redness and swelling at the immunisation site, irritable or may refuse food or develop a slight temperature. All of these symptoms can be relieved by giving Calpol.

Immunisation is a way of protecting against serious diseases. Vaccines contain a small part of the bacterium or virus that causes a disease. It works by causing the body's immune system to make antibodies. When the child comes into contact with the infection, the antibodies will recognise it and be ready to protect. The booster does are given to provide longer term protection.

# DtaP/IPV/Hib vaccine At 2, 3 4 month

### Diphtheria

This is a serious disease usually begins with a sore throat, quickly cause breathing problem and damage the heart and nervous system.

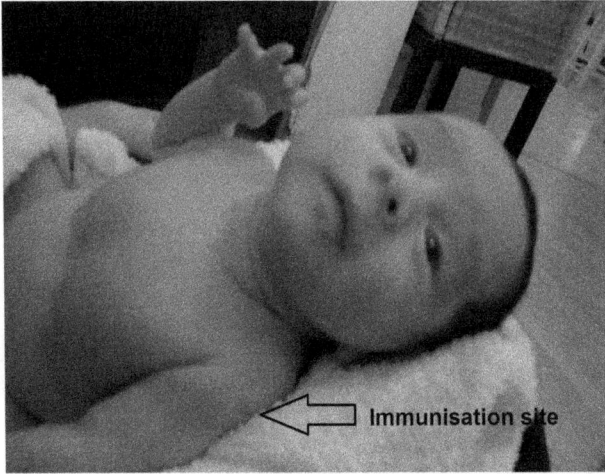

Figure 10.2: Immunisation site

YOUR CHILD WILL BE OFFERED THE FOLLOWING IMMUNISATIONS

| Age Due | Immunisation |
|---|---|
| 2 months | 1st Diphtheria, Tetanus, Whooping Cough, Haemophilus influenzae (Hib), Polio, Men C |
| 3 months | 2nd Diphtheria, Tetanus, Whooping Cough, Haemophilus influenzae (Hib), Polio, Men C |
| 4 months | 3rd Diphtheria, Tetanus, Whooping Cough, Haemophilus influonzae (Hib), Polio, Men C |
| 12 - 18 months | Measles, Mumps, Rubella (1st MMR)+ PCV · 12 and Hib + m cc |
| | 2nd MMR - usually at 3 - 5 years |
| 3 - 5 years | Diphtheria, Tetanus, Whooping Cough, Polio booster |
| 10 - 14 years | BCG after Heaf test |
| 14 years | Tetanus, Polio and Diphtheria booster |

Some babies will need Hep B and/or BCG vaccines. If in doubt discuss this with your midwife/health visitor.

Your health visitor or practice nurse will talk to you and give you written information about immunisations. This and other information is available on www.immunisation.nhs.uk and www.mmrthefacts.nhs.uk.

Do you know if you are immune to German measles (rubella)? If you are not immune you can be immunised to protect you and future babies.

Figure 10.3: Immunisation plan

# Tetanus

This is a disease affecting the nervous system, it can lead to muscle spasms and cause breathing problem.

Table 1

| When to immunise | What is given | Vaccine and how it is given |
|---|---|---|
| Two months old<br>17/10/2007 Gr | Diphtheria, tetanus, pertussis, polio and Haemophilus influenzae type b (DTaP/IPV/Hib) | One injection (Pediacel) |
| | Pneumococcal (PCV) | One injection (Prevenar) |
| Three months old<br>19/11/2007 Gr | Diphtheria, tetanus, pertussis, polio and Haemophilus influenzae type b (DTaP/IPV/Hib) | One injection (Pediacel) |
| | Meningitis C (MenC) | One injection (Neisvac C or Meningitec) |
| Four months old<br>17/12/2007 Gr | Diphtheria, tetanus, pertussis, polio and Haemophilus influenzae type b (DTaP/IPV/Hib) | One injection (Pediacel) |
| | Pneumococcal (PCV) | One injection (Prevenar) |
| | Meningitis C (MenC) | One injection (Neisvac C or Meningitec) |
| Around 12 months<br>19/0?/2008 Gr | Haemophilus influenzae type b, Meningitis C (Hib/MenC) | One injection (Menitorix) |
| Around 13 months<br>16/09/2008 Gr | Measles, mumps and rubella (MMR) | One injection (Priorix or MMR II) |
| | Pneumococcal (PCV) | One injection (Prevenar) |
| Three years four months to five years old | Diphtheria, tetanus, pertussis and polio (dTaP/IPV or DTaP/IPV) | One injection (Repevax or Infanrix-IPV) |
| | Measles, mumps and rubella (MMR) | One injection (Priorix or MMR II) |
| Thirteen to 18 years old | Tetanus, diphtheria and polio (Td/IPV) | One injection (Revaxis) |

Table 10.1: When, what and how to give the vaccine

## Pertussis (Whooping cough)

This is a disease cause long bouts of coughing and choking. This makes it hard to breath.

## Polio

It is a virus attacks the nervous system. It can cause permanent paralysis of muscles. In case of it affects the chest muscles or the brain, it can kill.

# Hib

It is an infection caused by Haemophilus influenza type B bacteria. This leads to major illnesses such as blood poisoning, pneumonia and meningitis.

It is quite normal after immunisation, the baby could be miserable and a small lump where had the injection.

Table 10.2: Primary course of vaccinations

# Pneumococcal (PCV) vaccine at 2 and 4 Months

This infection causes ear infections, pneumonia and meningitis. Colpol may help in case of mild fever after immunisation.

Born from Kidney Transplant Mother

# MenC vaccine at 3 and 4 Months

This protects against meningitis and blood poisoning caused by meningococcal group C bacteria.

Table 10.3: Meningococcal C vaccination

# Hib/MenC vaccine at 12 Months

This booster dose provides long term protection against meningitis and septicaemia.

# MMR vaccine at 13 Months

This protects against measles, mumps and rubella (German measles)

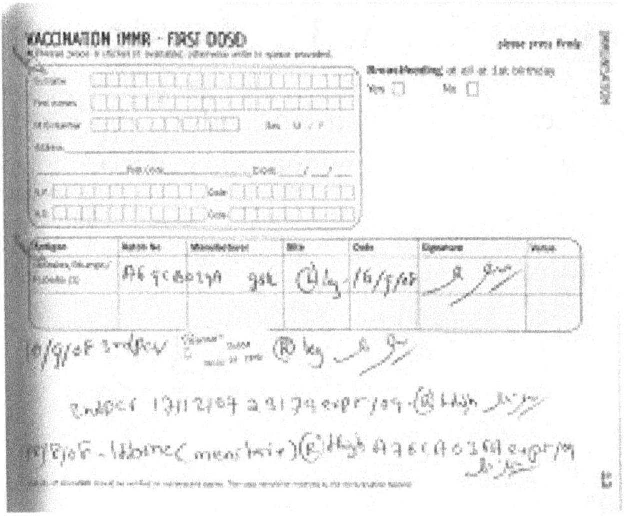
VACCINATION (MMR - FIRST DOSE)

please press firmly

Breastfeeding at all at 1st birthday

Yes ☐ No ☐

Surname

First names

Sex M / F

Address

Post Code

D.O.B. ___/___/___

| Antigen | Batch No | Manufacturer | Site | Date | Signature | Venue |
|---|---|---|---|---|---|---|
| Measles/Mumps/Rubella (1) | | | | | | |
| | | | | | | |

Figure 10.4: MMR first dose

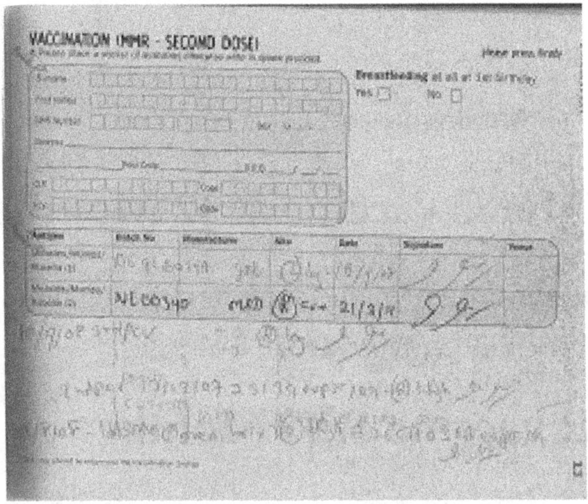
VACCINATION (MMR - SECOND DOSE)

please press firmly

Breastfeeding at all at 1st birthday

Yes ☐ No ☐

| Antigen | Batch No | Manufacturer | Site | Date | Signature | Venue |
|---|---|---|---|---|---|---|
| Measles/Mumps/Rubella (1) | | | | | | |
| Measles/Mumps/Rubella (2) | | | | 21/3/10 | | |

Figure 10.5: MMR second dose

## Measles

It is caused by an infectious virus, have high fever, a rash and unwell. The complications include chest infections, fits, encephalitis and brain damage. A cough or a sneeze can spread the virus over a wide area.

## Mumps

It caused by the virus can lead to fever, headache and painful, swollen glands in the face, neck and jaw. It results in permanent deafness, viral meningitis and encephalitis. It also can cause painful swelling of the testicles in males and the ovaries in females.

Table 10.4: Preschool booster vaccination

## Rubella (German measles)

It is a disease caused by a virus. It is very serious for unborn baby since it can damage sight, hearing, heart and brain.

Three different viruses in the vaccine act at different times. Six to ten days, the measles starts to work. Children may develop a fever, rash and go off food. Three weeks later, children may get mumps like symptoms. In the six weeks after the vaccination, children may get a rash of small bruise like spots. However, this needs to be checked by the doctor.

# Pneumococcal Vaccine (PCV) at 13 Months

This is a booster dose for long term protection against pneumococcal infection. This will not give the same time as MMR because it is overloading the immune system.

### BCG vaccine

This protects against tuberculosis (TB). TB is an infection affects the lungs, lymph glands, bones, joints and kidneys. It will give to baby come into close and prolonged contact with someone with TB.

| Vaccination | 2 mths | 3 mths | 4 mths | 12 mths | 13 mths | 40 mths | 13-18 yrs |
|---|---|---|---|---|---|---|---|
| Diphtheria | Part 1 Given on: 17 Dec 2007 | Part 2 Given on: 19 Nov 2007 | Part 3 Given on: 17 Dec 2007 | | | 1st Booster Given on: 21 Mar 2011 | 2nd Booster Due on: 16 Aug 2020 |
| Tetanus | Part 1 Given on: 17 Dec 2007 | Part 2 Given on: 19 Nov 2007 | Part 3 Given on: 17 Dec 2007 | | | 1st Booster Given on: 21 Mar 2011 | 2nd Booster Due on: 16 Aug 2020 |
| Pertussis | Part 1 Given on: 17 Dec 2007 | Part 2 Given on: 19 Nov 2007 | Part 3 Given on: 17 Dec 2007 | | | 1st Booster Given on: 21 Mar 2011 | |
| Polio | Part 1 Given on: 17 Dec 2007 | Part 2 Given on: 19 Nov 2007 | Part 3 Given on: 17 Dec 2007 | | | 1st Booster Given on: 21 Mar 2011 | 2nd Booster Due on: 16 Aug 2020 |
| HIB | Part 1 Given on: 17 Dec 2007 | Part 2 Given on: 19 Nov 2007 | Part 3 Given on: 17 Dec 2007 | 1st Booster Given on: 18 Aug 2008 | | | |
| Pneumococcal | Part 1 Given on: 17 Oct 2007 | | Part 2 Given on: 17 Dec 2007 | | Part 3 Given on: 16 Sep 2008 | | |
| Rotavirus | Part 1 Due on: 27 Sep 2007 | Part 2 Due on: 25 Oct 2007 | | | | | |
| Men. A | | | | | | | Part 1 Due on: 16 Aug 2020 |
| Men. B | Part 1 Due on: 16 Oct 2007 | | Part 2 Due on: 16 Dec 2007 | Part 3 Due on: 16 Aug 2008 | | | |
| Men. C | | Part 1 Given on: 19 Nov 2007 | | 1st Booster Given on: 18 Aug 2008 | | | Part 1 Due on: 16 Aug 2020 |
| Men. W | | | | | | | Part 1 Due on: 16 Aug 2020 |
| Men. Y | | | | | | | Part 1 Due on: 16 Aug 2020 |
| Measles | | | | | Part 1 Given on: 16 Sep 2008 | 1st Booster Given on: 21 Mar 2011 | |
| Mumps | | | | | Part 1 Given on: 16 Sep 2008 | 1st Booster Given on: 21 Mar 2011 | |
| Rubella | | | | | Part 1 Given on: 16 Sep 2008 | 1st Booster Given on: 21 Mar 2011 | |

Table 10.5: Vaccination program

## Hepatitis B vaccine

This protects against hepatitis B. It is given to babies whose mother is hepatitis B positive. It is passed through infected blood from mother to baby, Hepatitis is an infection of the liver caused by hepatitis viruses.

# Meningitis and Septicaemia Observation

It is important to recognize the signs and symptoms and know what to do.

Meningitis is an infection of the lining of the brain. Infection with meningococcal bacteria can also cause diseases such as meningitis, septicaemia (blood poisoning), pericarditis and arthritis (swelling of the joints).

Septicaemia is a very serious condition when the bloodstream is infected. The signs are cold hands and feet, pale skin, vomiting and very sleepy.

The main symptoms of meningitis in babies are moaning, high pitched cry, fever, irritable when picked up, drowsy, less responsive, bulging fontanelle, floppy, listless, stiff with jerk movements, refusing feeds, vomiting, pale skin, blotchy and turning blue.

The main symptoms of meningitis in older children, adolescents and adults are dislike of bright lights, vomiting, stiff neck (check by touch forehead with their knees), and bad headaches, fever, rash, drowsy, less responsive and confused.

The main symptoms of septicaemia in babies are unusual breathing patterns, fever with cold hands and feet, pale skin, blotchy, turning blue, shivering, vomiting, refusing feeds, red or purple spots do not fade under glass pressure test, pain, muscle aches, severe limb, joint pain, sleepiness and floppiness.

The main symptoms of septicaemia in older children, adolescents and adults are severe pains, sleepiness, less responsive, confused, cold hands feet, shivering, rapid breathing, vomiting, fever, stomach cramps, diarrhea, red or purple spots do not fade under glass pressure, arches in the arms, legs and joints.

It is important to get medical help urgently if the rash does not change the colour, fades and loses colour under glass pressure.

Born from Kidney Transplant Mother

# Chapter 11

# Screening for Premature

There are a series of routine health checks in the first few days of baby's life. This includes a hearing screen which uses two simple methods to check the hearing of babies. Both methods are completely safe and painless. Parents can stay with baby throughout the screen.

A blood spot screening test was done in the first week after birth. This is screened serious conditions such as phenylketonuria, congenital hypothyroidism, sickle cell disorders and cystic fibrosis. Early treatment can improve health and prevent severe disability or death.

## Blood Spot Screening

The midwife takes the blood spots by prick the baby's heel using a special device to collect some drops of blood onto a card.

# Phenylketonuria (PKU)

Baby inherits phenylketonuria (PKU) is unable to process a substance phenylalanine in their food. The baby with the condition can be treated early through a special diet. If untreated, it develops serious, irreversible and mental disability.

# Congenital Hypothyroidism (Thyroid)

Baby with congenital hypothyroidism do not have enough of the hormone thyroxine. It does not grow properly, can develop serious permanent both physical and mental disability. It can be treated with thyroxine tablets.

# Sickle Cell Disorders

This inherited disorder affects the red blood cells. It can change to a sickle shape and become stuck in the small blood vessels. This can cause pain and damage to the body, serious infection or death. The early treatment includes immunization and antibiotics will help prevent serious illness.

Carriers of sickle cell disorders are healthy and will not be affected by the condition. Other conditions such as beta thalassaemia major can be identified. In this condition, the baby does not make enough red blood cells and needs treatment for severe anaemia. The symptoms of sickle cell are usually anaemic, have a shortage of red blood cells, serious infection and damage to major organs.

# Cystic Fibrosis

This inherited condition affects the digestion, the lungs and have frequent chest infections. It can treat early with a high energy diet, medicines and physiotherapy.

# Screening Results

Your baby recently had a newborn screening blood spot test.

The test results were as follows:

| | |
|---|---|
| Phenylketonuria (PKU) | Normal |
| Hypothyroidism (Thyroid) | Repeat |
| Sickle Cell | Normal |
| Cystic Fibrosis | Not Suspected |

Please enter this result in your child's Personal Child Health Record (the red book) on page 24 (personal details). A copy of this result has also been sent to your GP and Health Visitor for their records.

Your baby's Thyroid test was normal but because they were born before 36 weeks gestation we recommend a repeat test after 13 Sep 2007. This will be arranged by your Health Visitor.

Figure 11.1: Screening blood spot test

If the results show to have phenylketonuria (PKU) or congenital hypothyroidism (CHT), parents are contacted before the baby is 3 weeks old, cystic fibrosis (CF), parents are contacted before the baby is 4 weeks old, sickle cell disorder (SCD), parents are contacted before the baby is 4 weeks old and refer to see a specialist. If the baby is found to be carriers, parents usually be told by the time the baby is 6-8 weeks old.

The Hypothyroidism (Thyroid) needs to repeat again because the baby was born before 36 weeks. Therefore, it has to re-test again four weeks later.

Your baby recently had a newborn screening blood spot test.

The test results were as follows:

| | |
|---|---|
| Phenylketonuria (PKU) | Normal |
| Hypothyroidism (Thyroid) | Normal |
| Sickle Cell | Normal |
| MCADD | Normal |
| Cystic Fibrosis | Not Suspected |

Please enter this result in your child's Personal Child Health Record (the red book) on page 24 (personal details). A copy of this result has also been sent to your GP and Health Visitor for their records.

Yours faithfully

Figure 11.2: Screening blood spot test (repeat)

# Thalassaemia Disorders

It is serious blood conditions affect the way oxygen is carried around the body. It can pass to the baby if both parents have the condition or both carry the condition. Healthy people who do not have the disorders can carry without knowing and carriers cannot develop the disorders.

The symptoms of thalassaemia are severely anaemic, need infusions or injection all time to prevent further illness and they need a blood transfusion every four to six weeks.

The antenatal pregnancy care can screen by blood test to check this order. They also need information about both parents' family ancestry who came from outside northern Europe.

In case of both parents are carriers or have thalassaemia disorder, the chorionic villus sampling (CVS) is a specialist test can do at around the 11th week of pregnancy. This uses a small piece of placenta to test in the laboratory. At 15th weeks of pregnancy, a small amount of amniotic fluid (Amniocentesis) is sent to a laboratory for examination. The results could show if the baby has inherited thalassaemia disorder, be carried or has not inherited. If the result is inherited, the doctor will discuss about the pregnancy, whether to carry on or ending the pregnancy.

# Newborn Hearing Screen

This screening test allows baby who has a hearing loss to be identified early. This is important for the development of the child. The support and information can be provided at an early stage.

There are some known factors may put a baby at risk of having a hearing loss, such as baby has needed special or intensive care in early infancy or other members of baby's family have had a hearing loss since birth or very early childhood.

Normally the screening test can usually be done before the baby leave hospital. The screening test usually done while the baby is asleep, does not hurt or uncomfortable, no anesthetic or sedatives are used.

A trained hearing screener or audiologist carries out the screen. There are two main ways of screening.

# Oto-Acoustic Emissions (OAEs)

A small soft tipped earpiece is placed in the outer part of your baby's ear. It sends clicking sounds down the ear. When the ear receives sounds, the inner part, the cochlea, produces a response an emission. The screener can see how the baby's ears respond to sound.

# Automated Auditory Brainstem Response (AABR)

Small jelly sensors are placed on your baby's head and the nape of the neck. The headphones are put over your baby's ears. A series of clicking sounds are played. A computer measures how the baby's ears respond to sound.

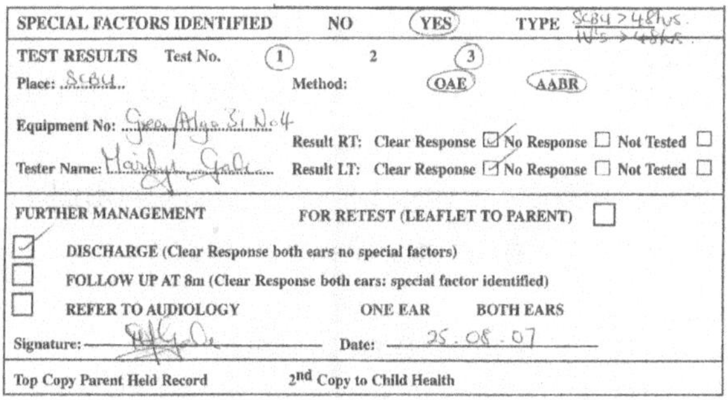
SPECIAL FACTORS IDENTIFIED NO YES TYPE

TEST RESULTS Test No. 1 2 3

Place: SCBU Method: OAE AABR

Equipment No:

Result RT: Clear Response No Response Not Tested

Tester Name:

Result LT: Clear Response No Response Not Tested

FURTHER MANAGEMENT FOR RETEST (LEAFLET TO PARENT)

DISCHARGE (Clear Response both ears no special factors)

FOLLOW UP AT 8m (Clear Response both ears: special factor identified)

REFER TO AUDIOLOGY ONE EAR BOTH EARS

Signature: Date: 25.08.07

Top Copy Parent Held Record 2nd Copy to Child Health

Figure 11.3: Hearing test

Since the baby born premature at 32 weeks and had to stay in the SCBU more than 48 hours and had IV's more than 48 hours. There is a special factor identified in newborn hearing screening.

If the screening test does not show a clear response, it may be because there is background noise, temporary blockage in the ears or the baby was not unsettled at the time of the screening. Therefore, it has to be tested again. It is about 0.3% of premature baby who has stayed more than two days in the intensive care has a hearing loss.

The screening tests show a clear response from both of the baby's ears. It means the baby in unlikely to have a hearing loss. The results show two checklists. The reaction is the sort of sounds the baby should react to and this sort of sound that the baby makes as he grows older.

# Checklist for Reaction to Sounds

Shortly after birth: startled by loud noise, blink, open eyes widely, stop sucking or start to cry.

- 1 month baby: starts to notice sudden prolonged sounds, pauses and listens.

- 4 months: smiles to the familiar sound turn eyes or head towards voice, show excitement at sounds.

- 7 months: turns immediately to familiar voices.

- 9 months: listens attentively to familiar everyday sounds and search for very quiet sounds made out of sight.

- 12 months: show response to own name, respond to "no" and "bye bye"

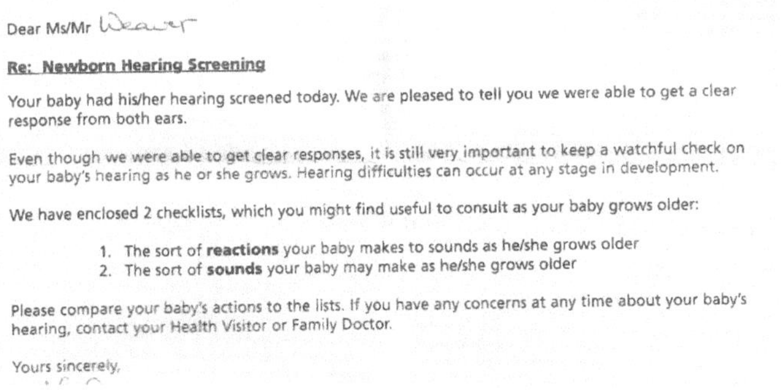

Dear Ms/Mr Weaver

**Re: Newborn Hearing Screening**

Your baby had his/her hearing screened today. We are pleased to tell you we were able to get a clear response from both ears.

Even though we were able to get clear responses, it is still very important to keep a watchful check on your baby's hearing as he or she grows. Hearing difficulties can occur at any stage in development.

We have enclosed 2 checklists, which you might find useful to consult as your baby grows older:

1. The sort of **reactions** your baby makes to sounds as he/she grows older
2. The sort of **sounds** your baby may make as he/she grows older

Please compare your baby's actions to the lists. If you have any concerns at any time about your baby's hearing, contact your Health Visitor or Family Doctor.

Yours sincerely,

Figure 11.4: Hearing test results

# Checklist for Making Sounds

- 4 months: make soft sounds when awake, gurgles and coos.

- 6 months: make laughter, singsong vowel sounds.

- 9 months: make sounds to communicate, babbling loudly; imitate sounds like coughing or smacking lips.

- 12 months: babbles loudly, use one or two recognizable words.

- 15 months: make lots of speeches like sound; use two to six recognizable words.

- 18 months: make a speech like sound with conversational type rhythm when playing; use 6-20 recognizable words.

- 24 months: use 50 or more recognizable words; put two or more words together, talks to self during play.

- 30 months: use 200 or more recognizable words, uses pronouns, uses sentences, ask questions and say a few nursery rhymes.

- 36 months: has a large vocabulary intelligible to everyone.

# Chapter 12

# Growth at Home

## Milk for Premature Baby

Since mother is a kidney transplant, therefore the baby cannot have breast milk. The post discharge baby milk formula is available on prescription.

However, it also needs need vitamin D and iron supplements. The baby should continue to receive this formula milk for 14-18 months.

The baby takes 70 – 110 ml of Nutriprem 2 seven times a day. This premature milk is on prescription and the pharmacy can support as a month basis. They are in a individual carton and ready to use. It needs a dry place to store this milks.

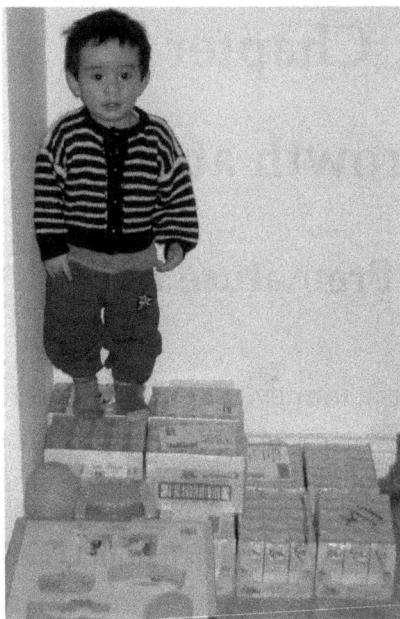

Figure 12.1: Premature milk Nutriprem 2 in monthly supply

About 18 months the pasteurized full fat cow's milk is introduced and changeover. The children's vitamins drop daily in cow's milk until around five years old.

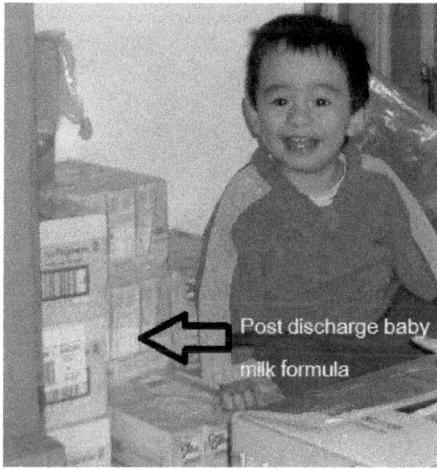

Figure 12.2: Post discharge formula milk for premature baby.

# Weaning for Premature Baby

Although giving premature baby milk early helps to develop the digestive system, it still may not develop enough to take solids. Thus, introducing the first solid foods when the baby is about six months or between four to seven months. If left till later there may be a higher chance of feeding difficulties.

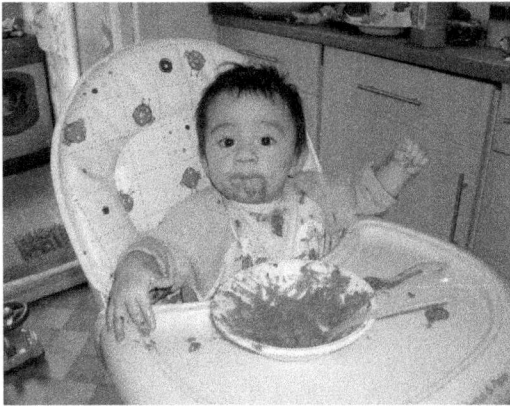

Figure 12.3: weaning

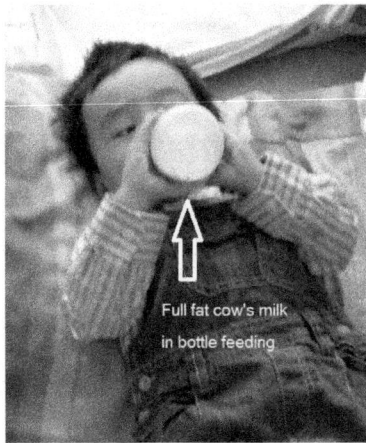

Full fat cow's milk
in bottle feeding

Figure 12.4: Full fat cow's milk

In addition, it may reach a point when formula milk is not enough to supply all the nutrition they need to grow well.

# Solid Food

Solid food is important for the development of mouths and jaws. Tastes and textures help encourage eating a good range of foods later on.

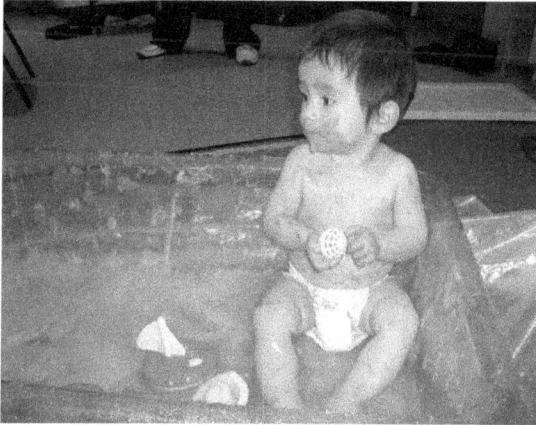

Figure 12.5: Messy plays

Introducing more foods and wider ranges of foods, increase the tastiness, improve the nutritional content of the diet and strong flavours such as meat, fish, lentils, peas, beans, butter, fats, cheese, puddings, yoghurt and fromage frais. The lumps should be offered by nine months. Once the baby starts lumping, it may also ready for finger foods.

Pure baby rice made with usual formula milk is the ideal first food, start with one meal a day. Fist food should be very smooth and runny. New flavours can be tried within the first week. Within one to two weeks, it can start to offer two meals a day. During the first month of weaning, milk should continue to be the major source of nutrition

# Self Feeding

Babies prefer to feed themselves and finger foods help to develop chewing and hand skills. After that the baby should be able to have family food by 18-24 months.

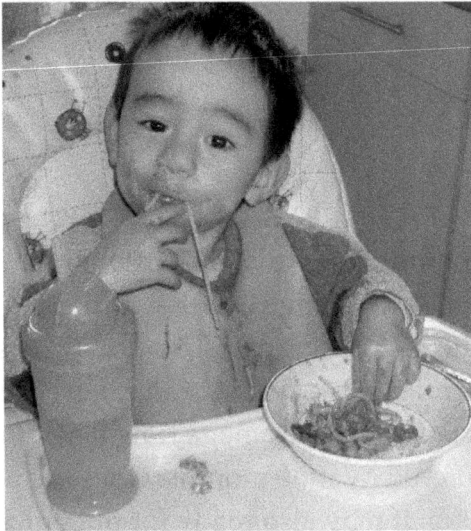

Figure 12.6: Food eating

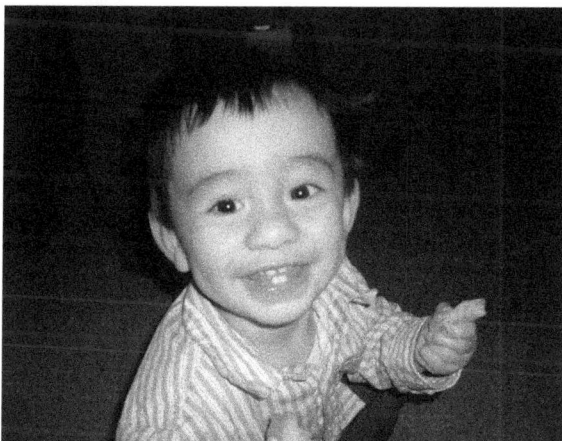

Figure 12.7: Self feeding

The signs that baby show ready for solid food when interest in other people eating, put things into the mouth and chewing them.

# Fingers Foods

Playing with food is an important part of learning about it and how to eat it. The food commonly associated with allergy such as eggs, fish, citrus fruits, nuts and seeds should not give until six months.

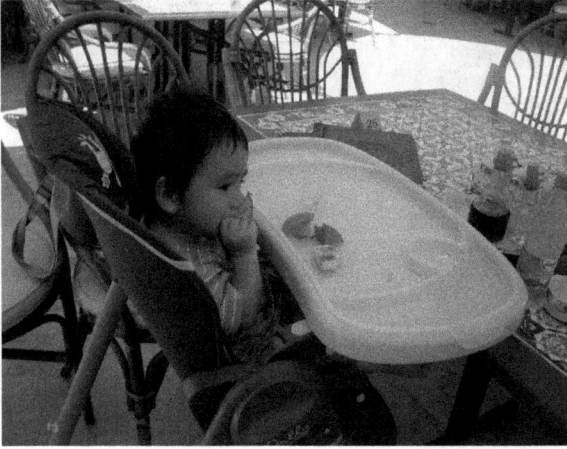

Figure 12.8: Finger foods

The whole nut should not give until the children age five years old because of the risk of choking.

Once the baby is on three meals per day, offer cooled the boiler water a cup at mealtimes. This is important, especially during hot weather to avoid dehydration.

# Water Cup

Start offering a cup around six to eight months and off bottles by 18 months. This prevents problems with the development of baby's teeth.

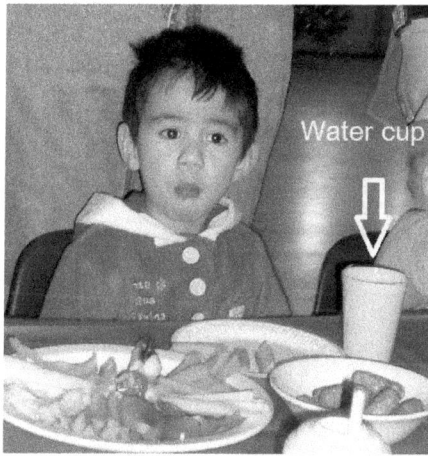

Figure 12.9: Water cup

# Baby's Teeth

Baby can start tooth-brushing before having no teeth, using baby brush and a very small amount of toothpaste. To reduce the risk of tooth decay, do not leave bottles of milk in the baby's mouth when sleeping.

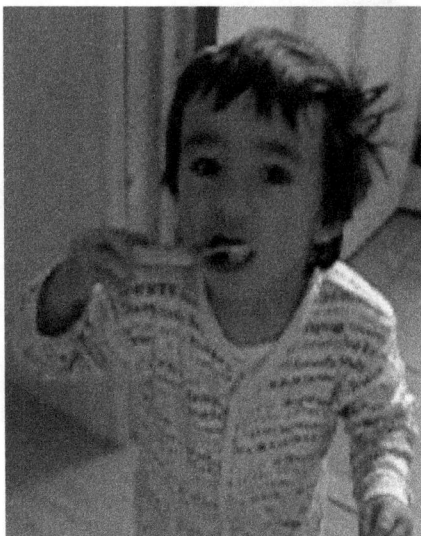

Figure 12.10: Tooth brushing

# Chapter 13

# Premature Growth

The best way to see how the baby is growing is by measuring weight, length and head circumference.

## Head Circumference

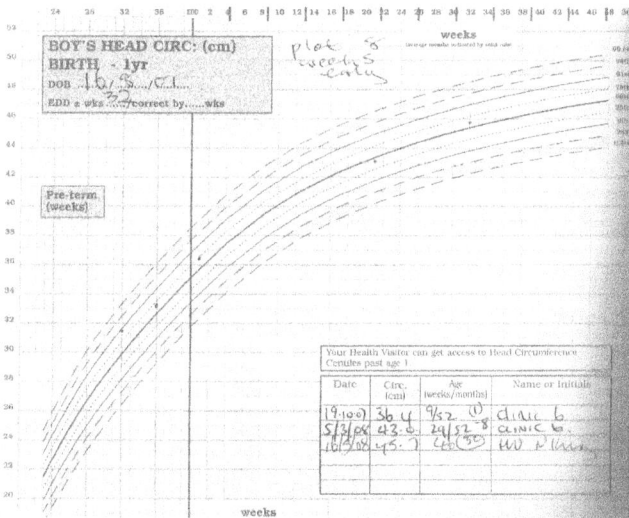

Figure 13.1: Head circumference measurement

Head circumference would be measured by health visitors. It should take from midway between the eyebrows and the hairline at the front of the head and the occipital prominence at the back.

## Weight

Your health visitor or doctor should fill in these boxes when they weigh your child and then plot the measurements on the appropriate centile charts.

| Date | Age (years/months) | Wt (kg) | Wt (lbs) | Name or Initials | Date | Age (years/months) | Wt (kg) | Wt (lbs) | Name or Initials |
|---|---|---|---|---|---|---|---|---|---|
| 16/8/07 | B1w 0 | 2.25 | 5lbs | | 27.12.07 | 19/52 ⑪ | 5.80 | 12.13 | HV |
| 4/9/07 | 2/52 | 2.58 | 5.11 | | 9.1.08 | 21/52 ⑬ | 6.07 | 13.6 | HV |
| 18.09.07 | 3/52 | 2860 | 6.5 | | 22.1.08 | 23/52 ⑮ | 6.40 | 14.2 | HV |
| 13.9.07 | 4/52 | 2.96 | 6.7 | HC 33.0 Nking | 5.2.08 | | 6.61 | | PHN |
| 19.9.07 | 5/52 | 3.26 | 7.3 | Nkang | 5.3.08 | 29/52 ㉑ | 7.02 | | CLINIC |
| 26.9.07 | 6/52 | 3.48 | 7.10 | Nkwd | 18.3.08 | 31/52 ㉓ | 7.28 | 16.1 | clb |
| 3-10-07 | 7/52 | 3.70 | 8.24 | Nkwd | 1.4.08 | 33/52 ㉕ | 7.40 | 16.5 | UA |
| 10.10.07 | 8/52 ⓪ | 3.96 | 8.11 | UA | 16.4.08 | 35/52 ㉗ | 7.81 | 17.3 | UA |
| 19.10.07 | 9/52 ① | 4.31 | 9.8 | clinic b | 1.5.08 | 38/52 ㉚ | 7.96 | 17.9 | UA |
| 24.10.07 | 10/52 ② | 4.41 | 9.11 | Gb | 16.5.08 | 40/52 ㉜ | 7.98 | 17.9 | NK |
| 30.10.07 | 11/52 ③ | 4.54 | 10.00 | UA | 1.7.08 | 46/52 ㊳ | 8.74 | 19.4 | UA |
| 6.11.07 | 12/52 ④ | 4.86 | 10.11 | HV | 12.8.08 | 51/52 ㊸ | 9.02 | 19.14 | UA |
| 13.11.07 | 13/52 ⑤ | 4.88 | 10.12 | UA | 10.3.09 | 14m2 | 10.65 | 23.5 | HV |
| 20.11.07 | 14/52 ⑥ | 5.06 | 11.2 | UA | 27.10.09 | 2ys 1/2m | 11.92 | 26.4 | UA |
| 25.11.07 | 15/52 ⑦ | 5.26 | 11.10 | Kg | | | | | |
| 11.12.07 | 17/52 ⑨ | 5.50 | 12.2 | UA | | | | | |

Head circumference, length/height measurements should be recorded and plotted on the appropriate centile charts.

Table 13.1: Weight measurement data

# Weight

Weight would be measured by health visitors. A self calibrating or regular scale would be used to weigh by infant and toddler. An older child would be weighed on a stand on scale.

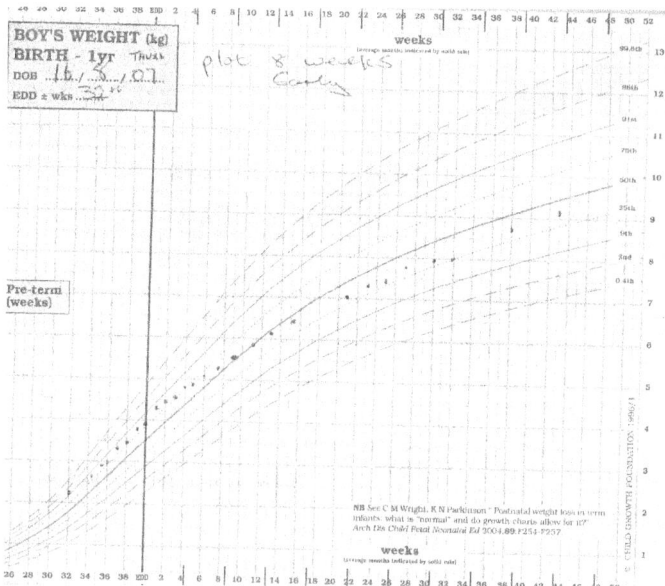

Figure 13.2: Weight measurement plot graph

# Infant Length

Health visitor would measure the length using proper equipment and technique. One person should hold the baby's head against a firm rest such as skirting board with the head facing upwards. A second person should bring a solid object such as the spine of a large book gently into contact with the heels. Then, measure the distance between the book and the skirting board with a measuring tape.

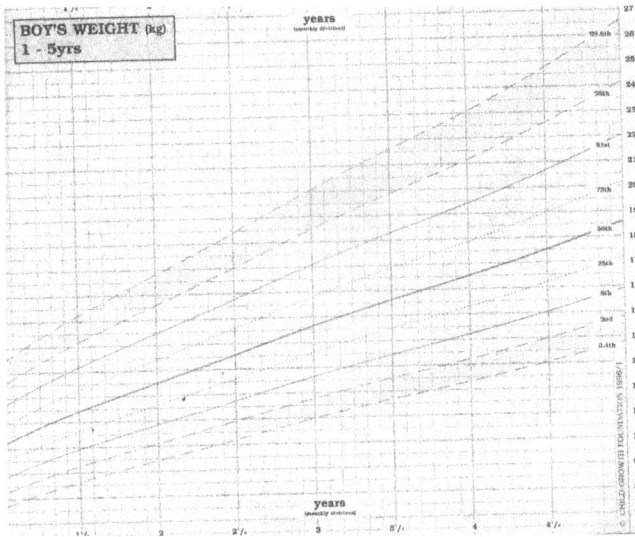

Figure 13.3: Weight plot graph 1-5 years old

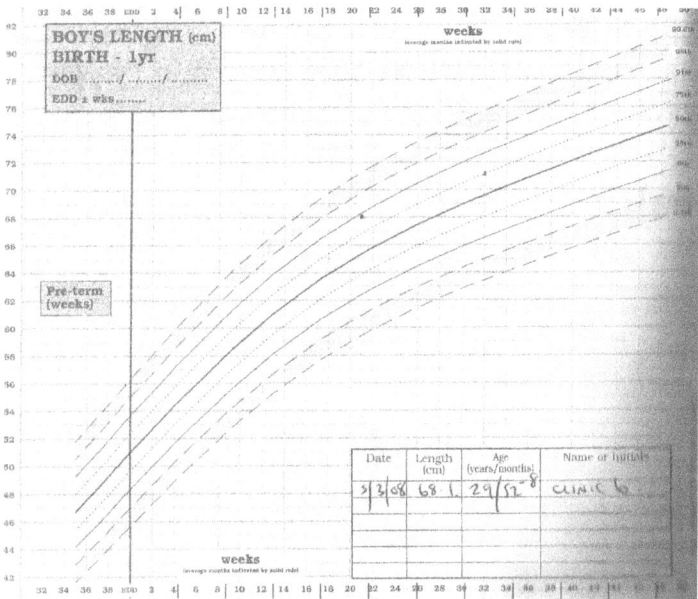

Figure 13.4: Baby length measurement

# Routine Reviews

Health visitors, consultants, specialists, GP, midwife and nurse aim to support parents in putting the needs of the baby. As part of their work, they offer routine checks and discuss the progress of the baby. The checks and reviews include checking the baby's hips, baby's heart, baby's eyes for cataracts, undescended testicles and dental checks.

Health checks and reviews are done picking up problems before they have been noticed. They plan and provide any other services the baby needs.

# Health Visitor

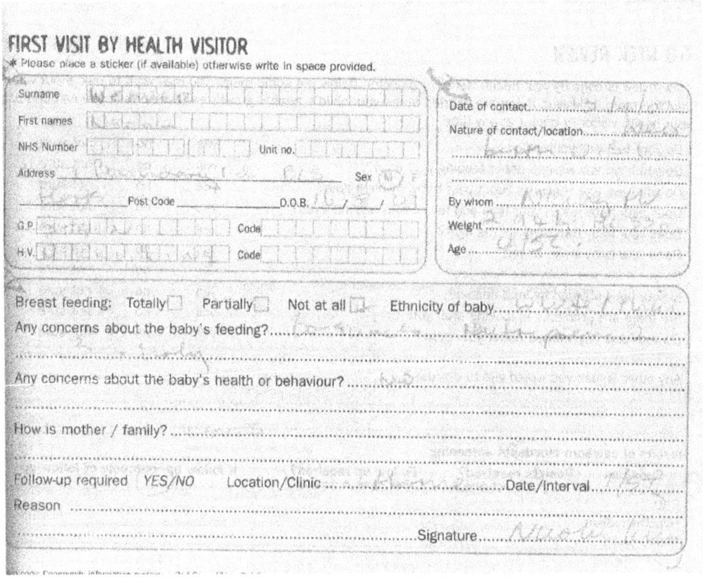

FIRST VISIT BY HEALTH VISITOR

* Please place a sticker (if available) otherwise write in space provided.

Surname

First names

NHS Number

Unit no.

Address

Sex

Post Code

D.O.B.

G.P.

Code

H.V.

Code

Date of contact

Nature of contact/location

By whom

Weight

Age

Breast feeding: Totally ☐ Partially ☐ Not at all ☐ Ethnicity of baby

Any concerns about the baby's feeding?

Any concerns about the baby's health or behaviour?

How is mother / family?

Follow-up required YES/NO Location/Clinic Date/Interval

Reason

Signature

Figure 13.5: Health visitor first visit

This is the chance to discuss any issues about the health and well-being of new baby such as feeding, sleeping, crying, immunization, child benefit, registering the baby's birth, health clinics and contacting the health visitor.

Table below shows record of any information about health and development weekly. This includes anything to discuss with the health visitor and GP.

| Date | Comments & any advice or treatment | Name & designation |
|---|---|---|
| 19/9/07 | Good weight gain. feeding Nutramen 2 70-90mls 3-4 hrly. Repeat guthrie taken for hypothyroidism. | Nursing H |
| 26/9/07 | Good wt gain - snuffly and feeling little and often review 1/52. | Nursing H |
| 3/10/07 | Good wt gain - still snuffly at night but back to routine at daytime. 110mls 4 hrly. | Nursing H |
| 10/10/07 | Has had a cold + now developed a cough. Discussed. No raised temperature. | |

Table 13.2: Record of baby health and development at age 4-7 weeks

# 6-8 Weeks Review

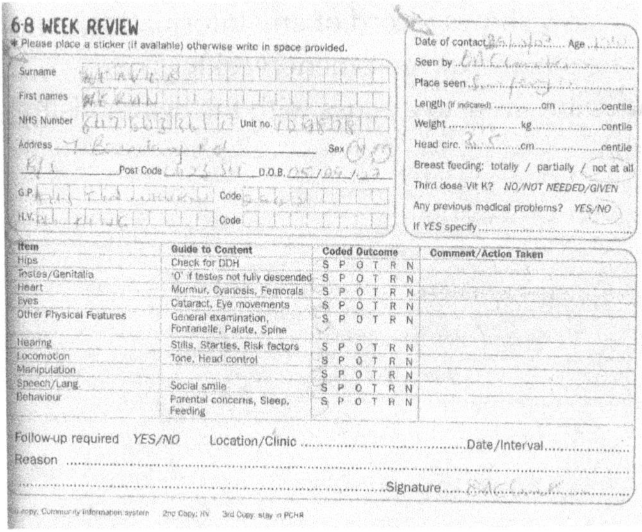

## 6-8 WEEK REVIEW
* Please place a sticker (if available) otherwise write in space provided.

Surname

First names

NHS Number ............................ Unit no. ....................

Address ......................................... Sex .............

.................... Post Code ................ D.O.B. 05/09/

G.P. ..................................... Code ....................

H.V. ..................................... Code ....................

Date of contact ....................... Age ...........

Seen by ...........................................

Place seen ...........................................

Length (if indicated) ...........cm ...........centile

Weight ...........................kg...............centile

Head circ. ...........cm.................centile

Breast feeding: totally / partially / not at all

Third dose Vit K?   NO/NOT NEEDED/GIVEN

Any previous medical problems?   YES/NO

If YES specify ...........................................

| Item | Guide to Content | Coded Outcome | | | | | Comment/Action Taken |
|------|-----------------|:-:|:-:|:-:|:-:|:-:|----------------------|
| Hips | Check for DDH | S | P | O | T R | N | |
| Testes/Genitalia | 'O' if testes not fully descended | S | P | O | T R | N | |
| Heart | Murmur, Cyanosis, Femorals | S | P | O | T R | N | |
| Eyes | Cataract, Eye movements | S | P | O | T R | N | |
| Other Physical Features | General examination, Fontanelle, Palate, Spine | S | P | O | T R | N | |
| Hearing | Stills, Startles, Risk factors | S | P | O | T R | N | |
| Locomotion | Tone, Head control | S | P | O | T R | N | |
| Manipulation | | S | P | O | T R | N | |
| Speech/Lang | Social smile | S | P | O | T R | N | |
| Behaviour | Parental concerns, Sleep, Feeding | S | P | O | T R | N | |

Follow-up required   YES/NO   Location/Clinic .................................Date/Interval............

Reason ...........................................

.......................................Signature...........................

1st Copy, Community Information system   2nd Copy: HV   3rd Copy: stay in PCHR

Figure 13.6: Health visitor review at 6-8 weeks baby age

At this visit, there would check for: Hips check for DDH; Testes/genitalia; Heart for murmur, cyanosis, femoral; Eyes for cataract, eye movements; Other physical features general examination, fontanelle, palate, spine; Hearing stills, startles, risk factors; Locomotion, tone, head control; Manipulation; Speech/Lang, social smile; Behaviour, parental concerns, sleep and feeding. There is required to follow up his health review when the baby at 40 weeks age.

| Date | Comments & any advice or treatment | Name & designation |
|------|-----------------------------------|--------------------|
| | Advised to raise head of mattress /cot | |
| | Ensure air is humid. If develops other | |
| | symptoms or parents are concerned, see GP | K.Whainwright. |
| 30/10/07 | clinic: _for_ _X_ _yesterday_ _(L)_ _sticky_ _eye_ | |
| | - spam drops - discussed use + use of mycostasis | |
| | clean eyes constantly - being seen | |
| | 1-2cps to saturate from - discussed review | |
| | + distance etc. Se "4p (Tig 100ru feb)" + EPC n v.o. | |
| 6.11.07 | Gained excellent weight gain this week, due to | |
| | change in routine. Chairman - has hypram | |
| | vetusing regularly, advised to use x 4 per | |
| | day - to clear nappies. | L. Mullins |

Table 13.3: Health and development record at age 8-9 weeks

# Neonatal Intensive Care Unit (NICU)

Previous problems of the baby was premature 32+6 gestation now corrects to term +1 week, Respiratory Distress Syndrome (RDS) –ventilated for 3 days, and Sepsis which is a common and potentially life-threatening condition triggered by an infection.

It is in NICU followed up clinically. The baby normal development as expected. BCG site has a positive reaction, feeding well, positive Moro reflex, heart sounds normal, chest was clear, abdomen soft and testicles were both descended into the scrotum.

Figure 13.7: Follow up at NICU

Table 13.4: Health review at 8 weeks baby age

# Ultrasound Kidneys

The premature baby was born from the kidney transplant mother. Therefore, the baby needs to have an ultrasound urinary tract scan at age 24 weeks to check his kidney functions.

| | | |
|---|---|---|
| For | : | **US URINARY TRACT SCAN** |
| | : | US KIDNEYS |
| On | : | **Wednesday 5th March 2008** at **2:20 pm.** |
| At | : | **Ultrasound Department, Level 3** |

We have received a request from your Consultant/GP, for you to have an ultrasound examination. This will take approximately half an hour and should not cause you any discomfort.

Figure 13.8: Ultrasound kidneys at 24 weeks

# 40 Weeks Old Review

When the baby reach at 40 weeks age, it is time to recheck grow matter, hips, fine mortar and eyes, etc. The thigh bones may be out of the hip joint. This is called Developmental Dysplasia of the Hip (DDH). There are some indications such as the baby drags a leg when crawling, one leg seems to be longer than the other, can hear or feel a click in one or both hips, the child walks with a limp, when change the nappy, one leg cannot be moved out sideways as far as the other leg and a difference in the deep skin creases of the thighs between the two legs.

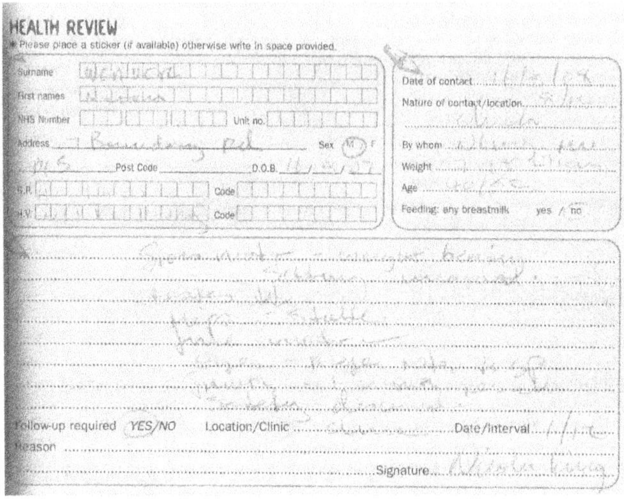

Figure 13.9: Health visitor review at 40 weeks

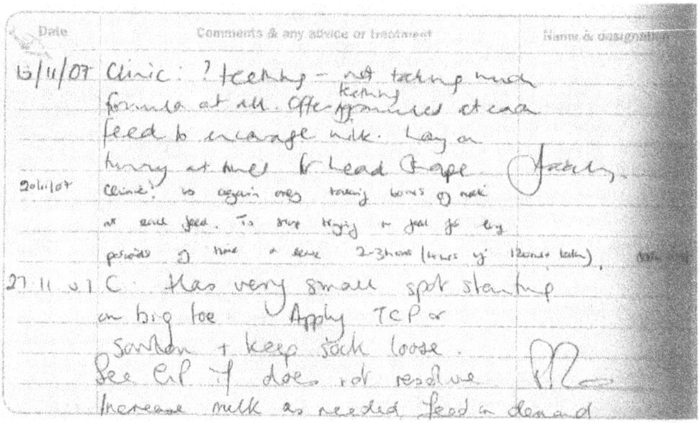

Table 13.5: Health and development record at age 10-12 weeks

Born from Kidney Transplant Mother

| Date | Comments & any advice or treatment | Name & designation |
|---|---|---|
| 27.12.07 | Anne Bottle feeding approx 120-140 mls per feed x8 per day, feeding more at night advised re routine - Maternal concern re illness - Checked symptoms NAD to see GP if no improvement | H V L Mullin |
| 22.1.08 | Clinic. feeding very chaotic during day but at night will feed readily + take approx 180-200ml each time. Discussed - try to feed undistracted during day + leave at least 3hrs between feeds. See 2-3 weeks. | NVRB |
| 5/2/08 | Clinic: baby has been passing blood | |

Table 13.6: Health and development record at 16-22 weeks

| Date | Comments & any advice or treatment | Name & designation |
|---|---|---|
| | in urine. Advised to see Drs at Addenbrookes - born very premature, in SCBU for 4/52. Own GP too busy to see | family |
| 5/3/08 | Attended for Neonatal F/U. Baby born on 9th → now on 6th. No feeding full intake should be ~1L/day in 6 feeds. Averages 600mls. Plan: liaise with HV re ↑ milk intake before adding in weaning solids | NICU Paed SPR SHO |
| 18/3/08 | Clinic: weight stable. Weaning commenced | |

Table 13.7: Health and development record at age 26-28 weeks

| Date | Comments & any advice or treatment | Name & designation |
|---|---|---|
| | - discussed progressing auto diseases | |
| | - using multi to mix. Apt to be made | |
| | for own H.V. | _(initials)_ |
| 1/4/08 | Clinic. Has had nappy rash, clotrimazole was prescribed. Now improved & needs to try Metanium cream to restore to normal. Started on solids | |
| 18/4/08 | Clinic. Satisfactory weight gain. Dry skin on arms + legs. Advised to apply aqueous cream to affected areas four times a day. Taking solids - to introduce 3rd meal. | R.Wainwright |
| 1/5/08 | Clinic. Sore nappy area. Has used various | |

Table 13.8: Health and development record at age 30-40 weeks

There is still a requirement to follow up his health review when the baby at two years to check if his development right at his age.

# 2 years old Review

Most of the premature babies will catch up to the baby born full term when they are about 2 years old age.

## HEALTH REVIEW
* Please place a sticker (if available) otherwise write in space provided.

Surname

First names

NHS Number                           Unit no.

Address                                        Sex

                Post Code              D.O.B.    /    /

G.P.                         Code

H.V.                         Code

Date of contact

Nature of contact/location

By whom

Weight

Age

Follow-up required   YES/NO    Location/Clinic                    Date/Interval

Reason

Signature

Figure 13.10: Health review at 2 years old

| Date | Comments & any advice or treatment | Name & designation |
|------|-----------------------------------|--------------------|
| | creams - generalised soreness ? allergic reaction to wipes. Advised re creams for nappy area & discussed use of water/ gentle wipes. Sore area behind knees, apply aqueous cream four times a day. | RSWainwright |
| 1/7/08 | Clinic. sore/ crusty area remains near chest. See GP if no improvement - to check ? squint. Not yet crawling but weight bears when held. | HV. NNeb |

Table 13.9: Health and development record at age 42-46 weeks

Dr. Kesorn Pechrach Weaver                                179

| Date | Comments & any advice or treatment | Name & designation |
|---|---|---|
| 20/12/08 | Nevan has chicken pox with red spots all over his body but he feels well. | Nevan Nevan. |
| 10/3/09 | ? Discoid eczema (R) upper cheek + (L) shoulder blade. Flared up - something weepy → GP for ? hydrocortisone cream. Toe-nail care - Advised | Kate Dibble HV |
| 27/10/09 | Clinic: sleep problem - try comforter crying. Relax when sonicky! ② Drinks milk ++, reduce amount, offer a beaker to encourage child food. | Nevan carn. |

Table 13.10: Health and development record at age 1 year 4 months – 2 years 2 months

The baby has his age appropriate development. There is no requirement to follow up his health review any more at the health visitor department.

# Preschool Review

When the child is at an age to start the pre-school at the age of two and a half years old, the school nurse would check the child health or development that may affect their education. Tests of eyesight and hearing are usually offered during the first year at school as well as general health assessment, including height and weight, speech and language, fine mortar skills, gross motar skills, social behavior, nutrition/eating habits, toilet

Born from Kidney Transplant Mother

training, sleep, immnisations, Playgroup, accident preventing road safety, passive smoke, dental advice, book start, children centers and sun awareness.

| Date | Comments & any advice or treatment | Name & designation |
|---|---|---|
| 15/1/010 | Clinic. 2y. development (2⅓/12) no | |
| | parental concern. Age appropriate | |
| | Book by given | 43    cohn. |
| | | |
| | | |

Table 13.11: Health and development record at age 2 years 5 months

The outcome is the child has age appropriate development.

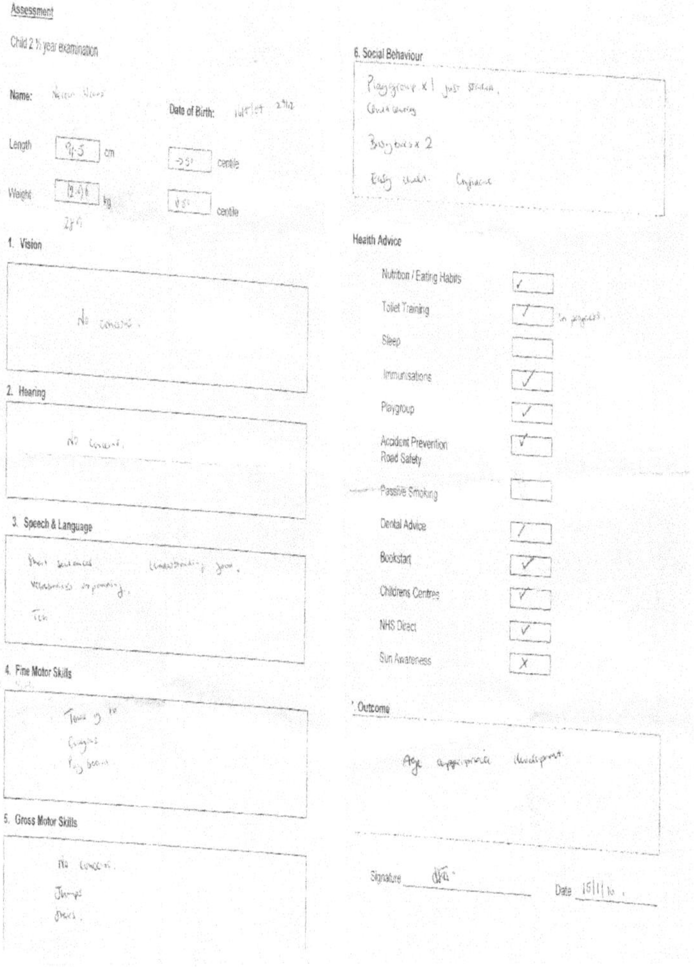

Figure 13.11: Child 21/2 year old examination

Born from Kidney Transplant Mother

# Chapter 14

# Mother Condition After

Unfortunately, complications of pregnancy are more common in patients who have had renal transplants, with early labour or delivery in perhaps 40% of patients and problems with fetal growth in 20% of patients. However, the chances of pregnancy resulting in the delivery of a health baby are so good.

As an experienced kidney transplant mother with three pregnancies result in one miscarriage, one stillbirth and one premature, this is a fighting not only with the body health but also the mental health. It was very difficult to discuss or talk about the loss.

## Learn from 2nd Pregnancy

The test results and inspection from the second pregnancy comes to be useful for the third one. It was clearly shown that a placental function had a problem. The week between 23rd and week 20th the growth of the baby fell from the 50th centile to the

5th centile. The blood flow pattern in the baby indicated that the baby was working hard to adapt to the poor nutritional supply. The baby was premature and small in size; therefore, the chance of survival if delivered would not be great. The doctors make a decision to watch and wait until the baby is 24 weeks before emergency delivery. Unfortunately, the baby's heart stopped just two days later.

In addition, mother's blood pressure become a problem in the pregnancy and required a small dose of Methydopa. Then, the blood pressure becomes an increasing problem. Therefore, the Labetalol was added. There were also features and Proteinuria that there might be an underlying pre-Eclampsia, which is common in patients with pre-existing renal problems.

# Mother Plan for 3rd Pregnancy

Since the mother, age of 37 years old, it should not postpone trying to conceive again for too long. However, it has to wait about 6 months for the blood pressure to settle down and off all anti-hypertensive medication before trying to conceive again.

The blood pressure medication has no effect on the future pregnancy, but the high blood pressure in pregnancy can affect kidney function in the long term.

Also, there is no concern about the effect of Tacrolimus, Azathioprine or Prednisolone on pregnancy. Thus, the pregnancy does not appear to have an adverse effect on the transplant kidney's function.

It is important to take Aspirin, 75 mg daily for 12 weeks until 36 weeks gestation in the next pregnancy to try and improve placental function. His blood pressure had to measure every two weeks, the aim for a blood pressure of <130/80. The kidney transplant pregnancy mother would be reviewed in the joint clinic between Perinatal Clinic and Renal Clinic every four weeks.

# Doctors' Plan for 3rd Pregnancy

The Perinatal Clinic, which consists of the consultant in Obstetrics & Gynaecology, Consultant in Fetal Medicine & Obstetrics and Consultant in Maternal Medicine & Obstetrics, plans to see the kidney transplant pregnancy mother at frequent intervals for close monitoring of fetal growth and assessment once more of uterine blood flow. They would plan to closely liaise again with the Renal Physicians.

The joint renal clinic would check the baseline renal function, full blood count and liver function. They would also arrange a scan at 16, 20 and 23 weeks.

# 3rd Pregnant Mother Condition

At around 16 weeks into the 3rd pregnancy, the transplant kidney pregnancy mother was well with blood pressure 106/66.The Creatinine was 93. This showed a progressive decline in the Creatinine over the last few months. The dose of Tacrolimus has been increased in the last week to 4 mgs twice a day.

The scan showed normal fetal growth. The uterine artery Doppler was also performed to see the likelihood of recurrence of intrauterine growth restriction and pre-eclampsia. The level of Tacrolimus would be recheck and back to the joint Nephrology perinatal clinic every 4 weeks. The blood pressure surveillance continues every week.

```
Dr : LEES C (Box 221)                                NHS No.:  6355 446 524
Wd : ROS221              WEAVER Kesorn                    DOB: 13/03/69
                                             Hospital No:      1662975
-----------------------------------------------------------------------
Spec : 1408:C00476R                               Rec'd : 14/08/07-1219
-----------------------------------------------------------------------
  Test                          Result    Abn   Reference     Units
-----------------------------------------------------------------------
  U/E
    Serum Sodium              |   136   |     | 135-145     | mmol/l
    Serum Potassium           |   4.3   |     | 3.4-5.0     | mmol/l
    Creatinine                |   127   |  H  | 35-125      | umol/l
    Estimated GFR             |    45   |     |             |
                       This patient has Chronic Kidney Disease Stage 3
                       (range 30-59 ml/min/1.73m^2; moderately reduced
                       renal function). If this is a new finding and the
                       patient is not known to renal services then routine
                       referral is indicated if there is :-
                       1. Suspected systemic illness (eg SLE)
                       2. Uncontrolled BP (>150/90 on three agents)
                       3. Microscopic Haematuria
                       4. Proteinuria (ACR >30mg/mmol)
                       5. Progressive fall in eGFR/raise in creatinine
                       6. Unexplained anaemia or other biochemical abnormality
                       Details at www.renal.org/eGFR/index.html
                       eGFR calculation assumes Caucasian origin
    Liver Profile
     Bone Profile
    Albumin                   |    29   |  L  | 30-51       | g/l
    Calcium                   |   2.08  |     |             | mmol/l
    Corrected Calcium         |   2.17  |     | 2.1-2.5     | mmol/l
    I.Phosphate               |   1.06  |     | 0.8-1.4     | mmol/l
    T.Bilirubin               |    5    |     | 0-17        | umol/l
    Alk Phos                  |   121   |     | 30-135      | U/L
    ALT                       |    13   |     | 0-50        | U/L
    CRP                       |    1    |     | 0-6         | mg/l
-----------------------------------------------------------------------

Department : Biochemistry   Tests : U/E, Estimated GFR, Liver Profile, Bone
```

```
Dr : LEES C (Box 221)                                NHS No.:  6355 446 524
Wd : ROS221              WEAVER Kesorn                    DOB: 13/03/69
                                             Hospital No:      1662975
-----------------------------------------------------------------------
Spec : 1408:C00477S                               Rec'd : 14/08/07-1219
-----------------------------------------------------------------------
  Test                          Result    Abn   Reference     Units
-----------------------------------------------------------------------
  Tacrolimus (FK506) Dimension |   6.6   |     | 5-15        | ug/l
-----------------------------------------------------------------------
```

Table 14.1: Creatinine level and blood test

# The Risk of Future Pregnancy

There were two concerns: Firstly, it is mother's age
and secondly past history and renal transplant.

From past obstetric history, the kidney transplant mother had a miscarriage followed by a pregnancy where the baby died at 23 weeks. This was associated with severe hypertension and growth restriction, and deteriorated renal function. Following this pregnancy, her blood pressure improved and she went on to have a successful pregnancy with a delivery at 32 weeks because of hypertension and deterioration in her renal function.

Unfortunately, there is a lower chance of conception and a higher chance of miscarriage and a higher chance of chromosomal abnormality in the baby.

With the kidney transplant mother current normal renal function and normal blood pressure, if she wished to have a further pregnancy, she would need to be monitored very closely. At some stage, it may be required to be hospitslised and almost certainly delivered early again.

The consultant in Maternal Medicine and Obstetrics have suggested the mother should start folic acid 400 microgram per day and take Aspirin 150 mg daily from about 12 weeks of pregnancy.

# Chapter 15

# Summary

The kidney transplant mother had been on immunosuppressant for her renal transplant throughout her pregnancy. The baby was born by elective Caesarean section at 32+6 weeks gestation due to concerns regarding the maternal renal failure.

The baby required CPAP within 5 minutes of life due to respiratory distress, had Apnea at 9 hours of age, was incubated and given a dose of surfactant, Benzylpencillin and Gentamicin. Since the CRP rose to 20 on day 2, he had a lumbar puncture; both blood and CFS were negative. He was on conventional ventilation for 3 days and was extubated on day 3 onto CPAP. He had been self-ventilating in air since day 4 with stable gases. His cortisol levels were normal and his blood glucose levels had been stable.

# Kidney Transplant Mother Summary

Method of Delivery: Scheduled Caesarean, Obstetric history: 0+2, Third Stage: Removed at Caesarean section in 7 minutes, Oxytocics: Syntocinon i/v (infusion), Pain relief: combined spinal and epidural, Placenta: condition normal and completeness, Blood loss: 500 mls, Pastpartum problem: Pregnancy induced hypertension, renal transplant, raised blood pressure and Creatinine.

## Mother Past Medical History

- Hypertension
- Kidney transplant
- Maternal renal pathology unknown

## Previous Pregnancies

- 23 weeks, Breech presentation Miscarriage
- Spontaneous Miscarriage

## History of 3rd Pregnancy

- PIH (Pregnancy-induced hypertension) which is a form of high blood pressure in pregnancy. The high blood pressure is chronic hypertension - high blood pressure that is present before pregnancy begins

# Antenatal Screening

- Hep B negative

- Rubella immune

- HIV negative

- VRDL negative

# Drugs during Pregnancy

- Tacrolimus

- Azathioprine

- Prednisolone

# Premature Baby Summary

Birth status: live birth at 32+6 weeks, Birth weight: 2259 grams (5 lbs), Resuscitation: Mask and valve ventilation, Apgar Scores: 7 at 1 min, 6 at 5 min, Mins to Reg Resp: within one minute, Special care: immediate Neonatal Unit admission for prematurity and 32 week baby admitted for ventilator support. Postnatal stay: 19 days, Feeding: Artificial, Weight change: 321 gram gain since birth, Bowels opened: Yellow, Umbilicus: Clean.

# Diagnosis during stay in Neonatal Unit

- Prematurity (32-37 weeks)
- Respiratory distress of newborn
- Sepsis Suspected

# Other Procedures

- Umbilical arterial catheter
- Umbilical catheter
- Lumbar puncture

# Delivery

- Presentation: Cephalic
- Mode: Elective section
- Liquor: Amniotic fluid clear
- Condition: Good

# Resuscitation

Baby cried immediately after birth, given facial Oxygen, grunting and nasal flaring at five minutes, started on nasal CPAP and transferred to NICU.

# Levels of Care

- 5 days of Intensive (Level 1) care
- 9 days of Special (Level 3) care

# Drugs given during a stay

- Benzyl Penicillin
- Gentamicin
- Furosemide
- Caffeine
- Dalavit
- Folic Acid

# Respiratory System

Diagnosis: Respiratory distress of newborn, 2 days of ventilation, 1 day of CPAP, had an episode of Apnea at 9 hours of age, was incubated, given one dose of surfactant, conventional ventilation for 3 days and was extubated on day onto CPAP, self ventilating in air since day 4 with stable gases.

# Neurology and Cranial Ultrasounds

Cranial ultrasound scans performed on day one, The result shows normal. There had been no neurological concern.

# Sepsis and Microbiology

Diagnosis: Sepsis Suspected

Blood was taken shortly after birth, started on Benzylpencillin and Gentamicin.

On day two, the CRP raised to 20 (which C-reactive protein (CRP) is a substance produced by the liver that increases in the presence of inflammation in the body), A lumbar puncture had preformed (where A lumbar puncture is a medical procedure where a needle is inserted into the lower part of the spine to test for conditions affecting the brain, spinal cord or other parts of the nervous system. During the procedure, pressure is measured and samples of Cerebrospinal fluid (CSF) are taken from inside the spine). The results showed both blood and cerebrospinal fluid (CSF) was negative. The baby received intravenous antibiotics for 5 days.

# Metabolic

Metabolic is the biochemical processes involved in the body's normal functioning. Risk factors are traits, conditions, or habits that increase your chance of developing a disease. As the kidney transplant mother had been on immunosuppressant for her renal transplant throughout her pregnancy. The baby's cortisol level where Cortisol, a glucocorticoid (steroid hormone), is produced from cholesterol in the two adrenal glands located on top of each kidney) to exclude adrenal suppression, all three random cortisol levels were normal and blood glucose levels had been stable.

# Gastrointestinal Nutrition

The baby was fed with Nutriprem 2 via bottles 3-4 hourly.

# Details at Discharge

Weight: 2140 grams.

Head circumference: 32.8 cm.

# Drugs at Discharge

-   Dalivit 0.3 ml OD until fully weaned or 12 months of age.

-   Sytron 1 ml OD at 4 weeks until fully weaned or 12 months of age.

# Immunisations

-   BCG immunisation dose 0.05 ml on left arm. The site of vaccination should be checked in 6 weeks.

-   Blood spot screening test 1 (protocol taken at day 5-8 of life).

-   Blood spot screening test 2 (to be taken at 36 weeks corrected gestation.

# Follow Up

-   At Neonatal outpatient clinic in 6 weeks.

-   In the neonatal registrar in 6 weeks.

# References

- A guide to the Premature Baby's Immunisation Program.

- Screening for sickle cell and thalassaemia in pregnancy.

- Newborn blood spot screening for your baby.

- A guide to immunisations up to 13 months of age.

- Newborn hearing screening program.

- Weaning your premature baby.

- Get well soon without antibiotics, European antibiotic Awareness day.

- Weaning starting solid food.

- Personal child health record, Royston, Buntingford and Bishop's Stortford, Primary care trust.

- The Rosie Hospital Maternity Services.

- Watching and Understanding your premature baby.

- Postnatal Care Record, Cambridge University Hospitals.

- Your Pregnancy Diary: When a baby is born, so is a mother.

- Screening tests for you and your baby.

- The Rosie Hospital, Patient Information: Caesarean section: A guide to Anaesthesia.

- Consent to a hospital post mortem examination on a baby or child.

- Information and support for the families of sick and premature babies.

- Transferring mothers and babies to other units.

- Where will you have your baby, home or hospital?

- Hyperglycaemia and outcome of pregnancy in Cambridge.

# Index

# PECHRACH PUBLISHING

You may be interested in other titles from Pechrach publishing:

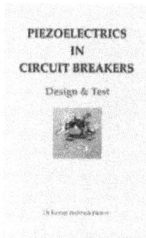

Paperback: 180 pages
Language: English
ISBN-10: 0993117805
ISBN-13: 978-0993117800

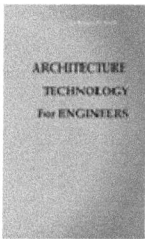

Paperback: 268 pages
Language: English
ISBN-10: 099311783X
ISBN-13: 978-0993117831

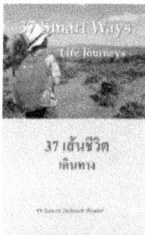

Paperback: 260 pages
Language: English, Thai
ISBN-10: 0993117813
ISBN-13: 978-0993117817

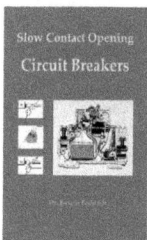

Paperback: 464 pages
Language: English
ISBN-10: 0993117864
ISBN-13: 978-0993117862

CIVIL SERVANTS
SALARY IN
THAILAND
History and Research

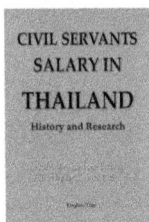

Paperback: 552 pages
Language: English
ISBN-10: 0993117856
ISBN-13: 978-0993117855

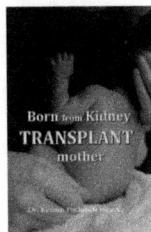

Born from Kidney
TRANSPLANT
mother

Paperback: 260 pages
Language: English
ISBN-10: 0993117848
ISBN-13: 978-0993117848

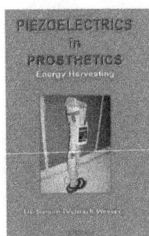

PIEZOELECTRICS
in
PROSTHETICS
Energy Harvesting

Paperback: 248 pages
Language: English
ISBN-10: 0993117821
ISBN-13: 978-0993117824

* 9 7 8 0 9 9 3 1 1 7 8 4 8 *